Voices
Neurodiversity

This groundbreaking A–Z of neurodiversity provides an accessible and definitive resource for professionals, families, and anyone seeking to better understand the vast landscape of neurodiversity as well as the experiences and potential of neurodivergent people.

Covering over 370 terms, the book offers a nuanced understanding of each term's multifaceted relevance and is structured around seven key categories:

- ❖ Neurodivergent identities, states, and models
- ❖ Emotional and mental health and well-being
- ❖ Social interaction, communication, and relationships
- ❖ Advocacy, rights, and community dynamics
- ❖ Support and therapy
- ❖ Education and professional contexts
- ❖ Harmful, pathologising, and stigmatising concepts and practices

Enriching this comprehensive reference, the book includes over 60 first-hand contributions from 12 neurodivergent individuals from across the world. Their diverse identities, lived experiences, and insights provide cross-cultural, intersectional, and deeply personal perspectives, offering powerful additional context to the definitions explored.

This encyclopaedia is an essential resource for neurodivergent individuals, professionals in social care, healthcare, education, and mental health, families, policymakers, the wider public, and anyone interested in learning more about neurodiversity.

Chris Papadopoulos is a neurodivergent academic, neurodiversity advocate, and father of autistic children. As the founder of the London Autism Group Charity, he combines lived experience, grassroots community support, and research to challenge traditional narratives. His work bridges academic insight with real-world support, making *Voices of Neurodiversity: An Inclusive Encyclopaedia* an essential resource for professionals, educators, policymakers, families, neurodivergent individuals, and anyone curious to learn more about neurodiversity.

Voices of Neurodiversity

An Inclusive Encyclopaedia

Chris Papadopoulos

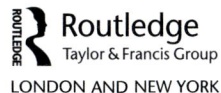

Routledge
Taylor & Francis Group
LONDON AND NEW YORK

Designed cover image: Getty Images

First published 2026
by Routledge
4 Park Square, Milton Park, Abingdon, Oxon OX14 4RN

and by Routledge
605 Third Avenue, New York, NY 10158

Routledge is an imprint of the Taylor & Francis Group, an informa business

© 2026 Chris Papadopoulos

The right of Chris Papadopoulos to be identified as author of this work has been asserted in accordance with sections 77 and 78 of the Copyright, Designs and Patents Act 1988.

All rights reserved. No part of this book may be reprinted or reproduced or utilised in any form or by any electronic, mechanical, or other means, now known or hereafter invented, including photocopying and recording, or in any information storage or retrieval system, without permission in writing from the publishers.

Trademark notice: Product or corporate names may be trademarks or registered trademarks, and are used only for identification and explanation without intent to infringe.

British Library Cataloguing-in-Publication Data
A catalogue record for this book is available from the British Library

ISBN: 978-1-032-76152-7 (hbk)
ISBN: 978-1-032-76154-1 (pbk)
ISBN: 978-1-003-47729-7 (ebk)

DOI: 10.4324/9781003477297

Typeset in The Sans
by Apex CoVantage, LLC

To my parents, for their wisdom, and my children, for their wonder

Contents

Introduction	xvii
About the author	xxi
Contributor biographies	xxiii
Understanding the seven thematic categories	xxxvii

A	**1**
Ableism	1
Absence seizures	2
Acceptance	3
Access arrangements	3
Accessibility	3
ADHD	4
Adjustments vs accommodations	5
Advocacy	5
Affective empathy	7
Affiliate stigma	7
Affinity cycle	8
Affinity therapy and passion-based therapies	8
Alexithymia	9
All Age Autism Guidance	10
Allistic	10
Allyship	11
Aloneness	11
Alternative assessment methods	11
Angelman syndrome	12
Animal-assisted therapy	12
Anomic aphasia	12
Anthropomorphising	13
Anxiety	13
Aphantasia	14
Aphasia	14
Appeals	14
Applied behavioural analysis	15

Apraxia	15
Art-based therapy	16
Articulation difficulties	16
Artificial intelligence and large language models	16
#AskingAutistics	18
Asperger's	20
Assistive technology	20
AuDHD	20
Auditory processing disorder	21
Auditory sense	21
Augmentative and alternative communication	22
Augmented reality	22
AuSocial	22
Authentic self	23
Autie	23
Autigender	24
Autism	26
Autism Acceptance Month vs Autism Awareness Month	26
Autism Act 2009	28
Autism parent	28
Autism spectrum condition	28
Autism spectrum disorder	29
Autism stigma	29
Autistic community	30
Autistic flow	32
Autistic inertia	33
Autistic language hypothesis	33
Autistic-led	35
Autistic-led identity support	35
Autistic-led mental health therapy	35
Autistic pride	36
Autonomous sensory meridian response	37
Autonomy	37
Autopia	37
Avoidant/restrictive food intake disorder	37
B	**39**
Behaviours that challenge	39
Binaural sound therapy	39
Bipolar	39
Body doubling	40
Brain-computer interfaces	41
Bruxism	41
Bullying	41
Burnout	42

C   45

Camouflaging	45
Care Act 2014	47
Celebration	49
Challenging behaviour	49
Children and Families Act 2014	49
Chronagnosia	50
Classroom adjustments	51
Code-switching	52
Cognitive behavioural therapy	52
Cognitive dissonance	53
Colour vision deficiency	53
Communication books and passports	53
Communication regulation partner	53
Communication through behaviour	55
Community spaces	56
Competency-based questions vs hypothetical-based questions	56
Complex PTSD	57
Concealment	57
Courtesy stigma	57
Cultural communication	58
Cultural competence	58

D   61

Deadnaming	61
Dedicated interests	61
Default mode network of the brain	61
Deflective masking	62
Demand avoidance	62
Demand sensitivity	64
Depression	64
Diagnosis	65
Diagnostic overshadowing	65
Dialectical behaviour therapy	66
Digital rejection sensitivity dysphoria	66
Digital twinning	66
Direct questions	67
Disability Discrimination Act 1995	67
Disability Living Allowance	67
Disclosure	68
Discrimination	69
Dissociative identity disorder	71
Double empathy problem	71

Dyscalculia 72
Dysgraphia 72
Dyskinesia 72
Dyslexia 73
Dyspraxia 73
Dysregulation 73

E 75
Eating disorders 75
Echolalia 76
Education Act 1996 77
Education, Health, and Care Plans 77
Educational advocacy 77
Educational psychologists 78
Ehlers-Danlos syndrome 78
Embodied identity 78
Emotional well-being 78
Empathic distress 79
Empathy 79
Employee resource groups 80
Employment advocacy 80
Empowerment 82
Emulation 83
Enacted stigma 84
Energy accounting 84
Empty phrases 84
Entropy 85
Epilepsy 85
Equality Act 2010 86
Eugenics 86
European Union Disability Strategy 2021–2030 87
European Union Employment Equality Directive (Council Directive 2000/78/EC) 87
Excoriation disorder 87
Executive functioning 88

F 89
Fake cures 89
Felt stigma 89
Fibromyalgia 89
Filicide 90
Fragile X 90
Functional neurological disorder 91
Functioning labels 91
Further education colleges 91

G   93
Global developmental delay   93
Gustatory sense   93

H   95
Hand flapping   95
Hate crime   95
Head banging   95
High-pressure socialising   96
Homeschooling   96
Human Rights Act 1998   97
Humiliation   97
Hybrid learning   98
Hyperacusis   98
Hypercontrol   98
Hyperempathy   99
Hyperfocus   100
Hyperlexia   101
Hyperosmia   104
Hyperphantasia   104
Hyperplasticity   104
Hypersensitivity and hyposensitivity   105

I   107
Identification vs diagnosis   107
Identity-first language   110
Illegal so-called 'cures'   110
Imposter syndrome   113
Inclusive design   113
Inclusive education   113
Independent or non-maintained special schools   115
Infanticide   116
Infantilisation   116
Infodumping   116
Inner monologue   117
Integrated care boards   117
Internalised ableism   117
Interoception   118
Interoceptive alexithymia   118
Intersectionality   119
Intrusive memories   120
Intrusive thoughts   120
Invisible disability   121

L   123
Language processing disorder   123
Late diagnosis   123

Learning disabilities and learning difficulties	125
Legal advocacy	126
Letter-boarding	126
Literal thinking	126
Loneliness	128

M — 131

Mainstream schools with SEN support	131
Masking	133
Mate crime	134
Media representation	135
Mediation	140
Medical model of disability	140
Meerkat mode	141
Meltdown	141
Mental Capacity Act 2005	142
Mental Health Act 1983	143
Mimicry	144
Minimally speaking people	144
Minority and intersectional minority stress	144
Mirror-touch synaesthesia	147
Misgendering	148
Misophonia	148
Monotropic split	148
Monotropism	149
Multigenerational trauma	150
Multiply neurodivergent	151
Music therapy	153
Myalgic encephalomyelitis	153

N — 155

National Strategy for Autistic Children, Young People, and Adults: 2021 to 2026	155
Nesting	155
Neuroableism	156
Neuroclearing	156
Neurocosmopolitanism	156
Neurodivergent and neurodivergence	156
Neurodivergent-affirming	158
Neurodiversity	160
Neurodiversity-aware curriculum design	160
Neurofibromatosis	160
Neurofuturism	161
Neuroharmony	161
Neurokin	161
Neurokin magnetism	161

Neurology	162
Neuronormativity	162
Neurophobia	162
Neuroplasticity	162
Neuroqueering and neuroqueerness	163
Neurospicy	165
Neurotypical	165
Nociceptive sense	165
Nomatnesia	166
Non-speaking people	166
O	**169**
Obsessions	169
Obsessive compulsive disorder	169
Occupational therapy	170
Olfactory sense	171
Oliver McGowan training	171
Online learning	172
Onychophagia	172
Outness	173
Overstimulation and understimulation	174
P	**175**
Panic attack	175
Parallel play and interactive play	175
Parent and family advocacy	176
Parkinson's	176
Peer advocacy	176
Peer education	177
Peer mentorship	177
Periventricular nodular heterotopia	177
Person-first language	178
Personal Independence Payment (PIP)	178
Pervasive developmental disorder-not otherwise specified	179
Phantom sensations	179
Phelan-McDermid syndrome	180
Phonological process problems	180
Pica	180
Polytropism	181
Post-traumatic stress disorder	181
Power of attorney	183
Prader-Willi syndrome	183
Precrastination	184
Prejudice	184
Premenstrual dysphoric disorder	184
Presuming competence	185

Procrastination	185
Professional stigma	185
Profound and multiple learning disability	186
Proprioception	186
Prosody	186
Prosopagnosia	187
Pseudobulbar affect	187
Pseudothymia	187
Psychological well-being	188
Psychosis	188
Public stigma	189
Pupil referral units	190
R	**191**
Reasonable adjustments	191
Regressive autism	191
Rejection sensitivity dysphoria	192
Repetitive behaviours	193
Resilience	193
Resource-based schools	195
Rett syndrome	196
Rhizomatic communities	196
S	**197**
Safe spaces	197
Saviour syndrome	197
Schizophrenia and schizoaffective disorder	198
Scripting	198
Selective mutism	198
Self-acceptance	199
Self-advocacy	200
Self-harm	201
Self-medication	201
Self-regulation	203
Self-stigma	203
SEND Code of Practice	204
Sensory assessments	204
Sensory avoidant	205
Sensory crisis	205
Sensory gardens	205
Sensory integration	206
Sensory overload	206
Sensory processing differences vs sensory processing disorder	208
Sensory rooms	208
Sensory seeking	208
Sensory-specific satiety	209

Sensory synergia	209
Sensory trauma	210
Shutdown	211
Six-second rule	211
Social anxiety	212
Social capital	212
Social communication	212
Social exclusion	213
Social fatigue	213
Social hangover	214
Social model of disability	214
Social Services and Well-Being (Wales) Act 2014	217
Social stories	217
Societal stigma	219
Somatic alexithymia	222
Special Educational Needs and Disabilities	222
Special Educational Needs and Disability Act 2001	222
Special Educational Needs Coordinator	223
Special interests	223
Special schools	226
Specialist colleges	226
Speech and language therapy	226
Speech dysfluency	227
Speech-sound difficulties	227
Spoon extending	227
Spoon theory	228
Stimming	228
Strengths-based approach	230
Structural stigma	230
Stuttering	231
Suicidal ideation	231
Sunflower lanyard	233
Synaesthesia	235
T	**237**
Tactile sense	237
Theory of mind	237
Thermoceptive sense	238
Tickertape synaesthesia	238
Tourette's	238
Transitions	239
Trauma	239
Tribunals	240
Trichotillomania	240
Triggers	240
Triple empathy	241

U
Unintentional stigma — 243
United Nations Convention on the Rights of Persons With Disabilities (CRPD) — 243

V
Vestibular sense — 245
Victimisation — 245
Virtual reality — 246
Visual processing disorder — 246
Visual sense — 247
Voiced empathy — 247

W
Wearables — 249
Wider autism community — 249
Williams syndrome — 250

Introduction

Welcome to *Voices of Neurodiversity: An Inclusive Encyclopaedia*. Whether you are a neurodivergent person exploring your identity; a friend, family member, or ally supporting someone; a professional in social care, healthcare, education, or mental health; or simply someone with a curiosity to delve deeper into the vast and fascinating world of neurodiversity, this encyclopaedia is here to provide you with critical knowledge and understanding.

Aims of the book

The primary aim of this encyclopaedia is to deepen readers' critical understanding and knowledge about neurodiversity and neurodivergence in an inclusive and accessible way. More than just providing information, it seeks to empower individuals on their unique journeys – whether through supporting self-discovery, enhancing the ability to self-advocate or assist others in advocacy, or nurturing professional development. By blending knowledge with practical and personal insights, the book aspires to be a valuable resource for personal growth, support, and professional practice.

The book aims to go beyond being a standard technical reference. Many of its terms are enriched with practical examples and real life narrative insights, designed to be both thought-provoking and emotive. The entries explore diverse aspects of neurodiversity and neurodivergence, including identities, well-being, relationships, advocacy, legislation, professional contexts, and more. As a work centred on neurodiversity, it also critically examines terms rooted in medicalised views of neurodivergence, so-called therapies, and other concepts that perpetuate stigma and harm for neurodivergent individuals. By doing so, the book challenges these paradigms and champions an inclusive and neuro-affirming perspective.

The contributors' stories

At the heart of this encyclopaedia are the powerful stories of its 12 contributors, whose diverse voices bring depth, authenticity, and humanity to its content. These 60+ narrative contributions transform the concepts into personal, moving, and tangible experiences, bridging the gap between theory and lived reality.

The contributors – neurodivergent individuals from different parts of the world, cultures, and backgrounds – have generously shared their stories to enrich this work. Together, their diverse identities and experiences create a tapestry of intersectionality that provides opportunities for deeper understanding and opens the door to further learning and impact for readers.

Their contributions are not only personal and profound but also instrumental in inspiring change and advocating for a more inclusive society. A heartfelt thank you is extended to each of these contributors for their generosity, courage, and willingness to share their lives with the world.

Visual accessibility

This encyclopaedia was designed with visual accessibility in mind. The A-to-Z format was deliberately chosen to streamline information and make it easily navigable.

To further aid navigation, each term is categorised under one (or more) of seven thematic symbols, which serve as intuitive visual anchors. These symbols group related terms and concepts, enabling readers to find information aligned with their interests or needs.

For example, those seeking concepts related to the emotional and mental health landscape of neurodivergence can look for the 🌱 symbol, while professionals interested in inclusive teaching methods and other forms of best practice can navigate to the 🏢 category. Please see page xxxvii for a full breakdown of the seven thematic categories, their meanings, and their associated symbols.

My own story

My journey into the world of autism and neurodiversity is both personal and professional, and I have dedicated much of my life to creating spaces where autistic and neurodivergent individuals can be their authentic selves and thrive.

My academic background is rooted in public health, with a focus on autism, mental health, and health technology. As a university lecturer, researcher, and commentator, I have sought to challenge stigma and advocate for inclusion. Over the years, I have had the privilege of contributing to projects that aim to reduce stigma and improve support systems for autistic people and their families.

In 2014, after my eldest son was diagnosed as autistic, I created the London Autism Group on Facebook to connect with other parents and build a supportive community. The response was incredible – it quickly became a lifeline for many families, including my own. But while the group provided vital support, I realised that meaningful, long-term impact required something more formal. So, in 2017, I founded the London Autism Group Charity, which now provides community, support, and education to autistic individuals and their families. Through this work, I have met countless incredible people whose compassion and insights continue to inspire me.

I also co-created *The Autism Podcast*, a podcast dedicated to sharing diverse autistic experiences, tackling stigma, and offering practical advice for navigating the world as an autistic or neurodivergent person. It has been an extraordinary privilege to amplify the voices of others and engage in discussions that challenge societal norms and inspire change.

This book represents one of the most meaningful projects I have ever worked on. My aim is not only to inform but to touch hearts, inspire empathy, and celebrate the richness of neurodivergent perspectives. I hope it serves as a valuable resource and sparks meaningful discussion and, most importantly, action that ripple beyond these pages.

When I am not working, you will find me spending time with my family, sipping a cup of Yorkshire Gold tea, or walking my two beloved cavapoo dogs, Cali and Cora. I'm also an unapologetic *Star Trek* fan and a lifelong supporter of Tottenham Hotspur Football Club – for better or worse!

Acknowledgements

The completion of this encyclopaedia would not have been possible without the unwavering support, guidance, and encouragement of numerous individuals. I am profoundly grateful to Venessa Bobb, Emma Dalmayne, Daryl Gordon, James Gordon, Katie Munday, Yvonne Odukwe, Simon Osborne, Georgia Pavlopoulou, and many others whose insights and feedback have been invaluable. Their contributions have enriched this work, ensuring that it is both comprehensive and compassionate.

Final thoughts

As you delve into the pages of *Voices of Neurodiversity: An Inclusive Encyclopaedia*, I encourage you to approach the material with an open mind and a compassionate heart. Let the contributors' stories inspire you, the knowledge empower you, and the insights motivate you to reflect on your own perspectives and take action in your personal and professional lives.

The journey towards a more inclusive and understanding world is ongoing, and each of us has a role to play. Together, we can advance the acceptance of neurodiversity, celebrating the diversity of human experience and building a society that uplifts and values every individual.

Contact information

You can contact me through the London Autism Group Charity at contact@londonautismgroupcharity.org. Or you can visit the charity's website at londonautismgroupcharity.org.

About the author

Chris Papadopoulos is a neurodivergent academic, neurodiversity advocate, and father of autistic children. With a career in academia and research, he has developed expertise in autism, mental health, and community health. He is also the founder and lead of the London Autism Group Charity, dedicated to supporting autistic individuals and their families.

Drawing from academic expertise, extensive charitable work, and lived experience, Papadopoulos offers a nuanced perspective on neurodiversity. His work bridges the gap between research, advocacy, and real-world support, ensuring this encyclopaedia is both insightful and deeply relevant to real-world challenges. In *Voices of Neurodiversity: An Inclusive Encyclopaedia*, he brings together diverse perspectives to create an accessible and comprehensive guide.

Developed in collaboration with neurodivergent people from across the world, this encyclopaedia explores the richness of neurodiversity in an engaging and accessible way. Through his research, advocacy, and personal experience, Papadopoulos ensures this work is both informative and deeply human, making it an invaluable resource for professionals, educators, policymakers, families, neurodivergent individuals, and anyone curious to learn more about neurodiversity.

Contributor biographies

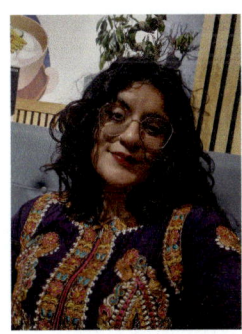

Iqra Babar

I am a 25-year-old AuDHDer (autistic and ADHD), Muslim, and Pakistani digital artist, activist, educator, and teacher based in London. I graduated with first class honours in primary education with qualified teaching status and have a keen interest in history, the humanities, and decolonisation in education. Currently, I am pursuing a master's degree in education at University College London. My academic interests include neurodivergent-affirming practices in education and envisioning a non-pathologising paradigm within the teaching field.

I was diagnosed as AuDHD at 17, during my final year of sixth form. Since then, it has been an enlightening and educational experience, helping me to better understand neurodivergent identities and, ultimately, myself. Alongside my studies and teaching, I pursue digital art as a passion. Through my art, I explore my South Asian culture and heritage, often through original characters and culturally thematic pieces. I am deeply interested in the intersections of identity, particularly around disability, neurodivergence, and the significance of media representation.

My work as an artist and advocate has led me to collaborate with organisations like the British Library on projects such as The Character Creation Zone: Create Your Own Comic Book Character. Additionally, I've contributed articles to platforms like Amaliah and MVSLIM, writing about topics such as navigating friendships as a neurodivergent Muslim and introducing Islam and disability acceptance. I've appeared on podcasts, too, including BBC Radio 4's *Beyond Belief: Autism and Faith*, where I discussed the intersection of neurodivergence and faith.

I am also the creator of the dark-fantasy webseries *DARJIN*, a vibrant story that explores themes of identity, culture, and neurodivergence with emotional and philosophical undertones. You can learn more about it at https://www.wattpad.com/story/365236065-darjin.

You can explore more of my work via my Linktree at https://linktr.ee/iqradraws.

Ben Breaux

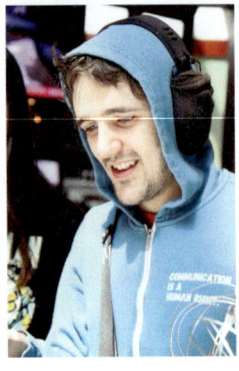

I am Ben Breaux – a 24-year-old nonspeaking autistic with epilepsy from Northern Virginia in the United States. I have written many articles for numerous autism and disability advocacy groups both in the United States and worldwide, and I am a very proud representative for my community on several advocacy boards and committees, both in the state of Virginia and nationally. I am currently working towards getting a full academic high school diploma via ACCESS, an online academic and support program for alternative learners. I strive daily to show the world that an intellectual disability will not hold me – or others like me – back.

My interests include elephants, chocolate pudding, and cheese. I also love the show *Friends*. I don't do sports on teams or anything, but I do like to dance. I like pop music, especially Whitney Houston and anything upbeat really. I have gone through a few phases of listening to all sorts of music. I like history and math the most in school . . . and writing, obviously, as I am pursuing a career in journalism. I have a white, goofy dog named Beaux. He's super fluffy and playful. I love YouTube, but I don't have a favorite YouTuber. I prefer to scroll and watch any random music or sensory video that catches my eye.

When I was a toddler, I could speak. I could have real conversations about all kinds of topics with all kinds of people. My mom said I had advanced language use for my age. I don't remember particular words I said, as there were really so many. And then there weren't – at all. When I turned 3, my life started to change drastically. I began to have limited speech out loud. Because I couldn't speak, I was suddenly seen as 'non-thinking.' No longer did people regard me worthy of a true education. It made me feel like I'd been mislabeled and discarded by society. During this time, I continued to teach myself all kinds of things by observing the environment around me intensely. No one knew I was learning this information. It was all stuck inside me. This went on for about 10 years before I started letterboarding.

I feel it is of utmost importance that non-, minimal-, and unreliably speaking autistics have equal rights, opportunities, and voices in society. So often do people with autism face stigma and hardships. We – as a community – must fight to be heard! It seems that most people do not see or comprehend that autistics can be normal people. So many hearts don't receive the support they need. I hope to adopt a new method of reaching out to this population through my contribution to this encyclopaedia.

Agustina Cardoso

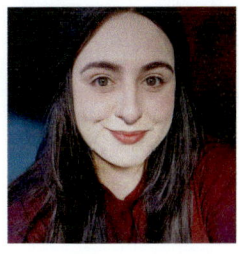

I'm Agustina Cardoso, a proudly autistic and ADHD graphic designer, psychology student, peer supporter, and writer behind *The Autistic Life*. Being neurodivergent myself, I've built a community that celebrates and amplifies the voices of people like me through thoughtful graphic design, educational resources, and storytelling.

Born and raised in Uruguay, my South American heritage plays a significant role in how I connect with others, bringing a rich perspective to my work. I'm currently pursuing a master's degree in clinical neuropsychology, deepening my understanding of the brain and further enriching my work in supporting the neurodivergent community. My lived experiences as an ADHD and autistic person shape everything I do, allowing me to express the complexities and beauty of neurodivergent life in a way that feels both personal and meaningful.

I'm passionate about creating spaces where neurodivergent individuals feel seen, valued, and supported. Through *The Autistic Life*, I aim to spark conversations that are often overlooked, weaving them into designs and resources that bring these stories to life.

In the future, I hope to establish therapeutic spaces where neurodivergent people can build skills, connect with others, and fully embrace their identities. My mission is to inspire change, foster understanding, and celebrate neurodivergence as an essential part of the human experience.

Joris Fouet

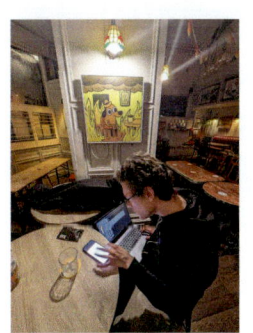

I was born to an intellectual family in France. We were all working very hard towards my success in the fiercely competitive French engineering schools. Academic performance seemed the only metric. And we were doing very well!

Also, I was miserable. Fighting against my whole body the whole time. It just wouldn't oblige.

I would regularly spend the whole night awake in my bed. I would bite my nails to the blood. Mere suggestions of failure would trigger acute asthma attacks. Those disappeared overnight when I found cannabis.

So I was a junkie. I could deal with that.

Somehow I still managed to find mentors, to power through the weaknesses and the haze, to reach their standards, at least to their satisfaction, definitely not mine.

I could never manage without compromising something, but I prioritised those carefully to optimise the scores.

And still, trying until they wouldn't let me.

And I did it! I got accepted into a prestigious school! I was set!

With just a little more work, I could have the sweet scientific career we always dreamed of. The one I could see my older peers and teachers making themselves even more miserable over. Wait, what?

There were also rockstars that had all the things. But they seemed to get it from draining the people like me in their environment.

I could push myself through it. But I was the only one left doing the pushing: family goals had been reached. Suddenly left to my own devices, one thing was sure, I was having none of that.

So . . . cannabis! Then music. Then I got kicked out of school. Then more music.

Having tried to find something to do in school besides studying, I landed on clubbing, discovering at the same time the trance of dancing, the anonymity of crowds, and the relief of purposeful sensory overloading. There was solace outside of drugs. Who would have thought art could help?

I started DJing. I was bad at it for a long while, then I was good. And after mastery came passion. Plus, I liked performing: people would come talk to me! I no longer needed to figure out the other way around.

I also took a job as a programmer, since I knew programming and needed the money. Well, corporate politics sure made me regret academic competition. I looked the part in the Parisian subway, but I kept being played in this new game.

After a couple of years, it became clear that I would only ever thrive in a startup. When there's two persons for a job, none of them has incentive to work harder than the other. When you have two jobs per person . . . do your job.

And the best I can do is a good job. Which I was told could be surprisingly good. But it would only happen in very specific, adjusted environments. And since it's hard to find a company that'll let you make your own hours, I had to start my own.

A friend had a good idea. I quit my job, swore I would never wear a suit again, and moved to Berlin to prototype on his couch. What did I have to lose?

I failed a few startups until I didn't. Turns out there is good money in counting things. One project took off in London. I moved there. Why not? At least they respect a good queue.

Throughout, the one and only thing that mattered was performance. In its name, I started meditating. I started journaling. And slowly I started hearing what I was yelling at myself. I went to therapy. We were just extinguishing fires. But it let me work better.

Until a new therapist brought up autism and wouldn't let me deflect. So I started reading up on it. The brain behaviour, not the social cliché. And finally, my life got explained to me.

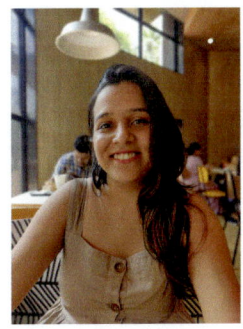

Aditi Gangrade

I've always been drawn to stories – how they connect us, how they shape us, and how they can change the world. As an autistic ADHD woman navigating a neurotypical world, I've lived through the complexities of feeling like an outsider, questioning where I belong, and discovering the power of community. Growing up in India, I often found myself searching for reflections of people like me in the stories around me, only to realize they were painfully absent. This absence, however, ignited a spark that led me to co-found Much Much Media and its inclusive original content vertical, Much Much Spectrum.

At Much Much Spectrum, my work and life partner Aalap and I are building something extraordinary with one aim: becoming the world's largest repository of content centered on social storytelling – stories of neurodiversity, disability, LGBTQIA+, and many other underrepresented communities. With over 75,000 people in our growing community, our platform is more than just a space for content – it's a home to the wholesome. It's where stories of resilience, joy, and authenticity thrive, creating ripple effects that challenge societal biases and redefine 'normal.'

I often describe our work as "social impact storytelling," but it's much more personal than that. As a filmmaker, I've directed short documentaries that highlight neurodivergent and disabled individuals, ensuring their stories are told with authenticity and care. Our filmmaking processes are neurodiversity-affirming, trauma-informed, and rooted in consent – because representation is not just about being seen but being seen right.

Growing up in a collectivist culture like India's, I understood the importance of community early on. But I also knew the loneliness of not fitting in. That's why

Much Much Spectrum isn't just a company to me – it's a mission. It's a space where people like me, like us, can come together, find connection, and celebrate our differences. Whether we're creating content, consulting with organizations, or collaborating on initiatives, our goal is simple: to make inclusion visible and actionable.

On a personal level, my identity as an autistic ADHD person profoundly shapes how I think and create. I'm deeply curious, fiercely empathetic, and endlessly committed to breaking down the norms that hold us back. Through Much Much Spectrum, I've found a way to channel my lived experiences into meaningful work – work that doesn't just represent neurodivergent people but empowers them to thrive.

When I'm not working, you'll likely find me baking something guilt-free for my loved ones – because nourishing others brings me a sense of joy. I'm a great listener (or so my friends say) and someone who finds endless fascination in the world around me. I treasure my small but deeply meaningful circle of loved ones and take immense pride in caring for them. They're my safe space and constant reminder of what matters most.

One of my proudest moments was directing the films closest to my heart, *Unmasking Autism* and *Parenting and Autism* – projects that have received love from across the globe. My efforts come from the belief that good representation has the power to change lives. If young Aditi had seen stories like the ones we tell, she might have felt a little less like an imposter and a lot more like she belonged.

As a Gen-Z entrepreneur and filmmaker, I'm not just creating content – I'm building bridges. Between the neurodivergent and neurotypical worlds. Between marginalized communities and the spaces that have ignored them. Between what is and what could be.

Ginny Grant

I'm Virginia (Ginny) Grant (she/her), a 40-something neurodivergent woman living on Gadigal and Wangal land in Sydney, Australia. As a parent of two autistic children, I discovered that I shared many of their atypical traits, leading to my formal autism diagnosis at the age of 39.

My Autism identification was a pivotal moment in my life. Looking back on my experiences through the lens of Autism, so much finally made sense. I embraced identity-first language immediately because I knew Autism wasn't just an 'added accessory' – it's an integral part of who I am.

Before my diagnosis, I spent years listening to a wide variety of autistic voices in the community. After my own identification, I felt inspired to share my voice, too. I've had the privilege of speaking and writing across numerous platforms, including appearing as a guest with Dr Chris Papadopoulos on the London Autism Group Charity's *The Autism Podcast* (episode 26) and hosting two seasons of Reframing Autism's podcast, *Amplified*.

More recently, I've begun to identify not just as autistic but as neurodivergent, recognising that a range of neurodevelopmental differences and mental health conditions influence how I think, feel, process, communicate, and socialise. My experience as someone whose neurocognitive functioning diverges from the norm is not about being 'less' – it's about embracing the diversity of human brains.

In my working life, I've been fortunate to follow my passions for books and writing. I've worked for many years as a book editor, helping to create children's and adult books across a variety of subjects. I'm also the author of *Australia's Greatest Landmarks and Locations* (2014) and have contributed to several other publications. Outside of work, my passions include animals, travel, and learning foreign languages.

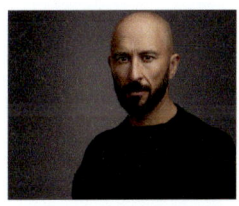

Andrew Kingslow

I'm a music producer and composer currently living in London. I first picked up music at the age of 4, grabbing my older sister's guitar and teaching myself nursery rhymes by ear. The sounds and patterns fascinated me. In fact, patterns in general captivated me – Rubik's Cubes, computer programming, and so on.

From ages 5 to 7, I had to wear an eye patch due to amblyopia (a vision issue where one eye becomes weaker than the other). Teachers thought I was a little slow to learn as a result. When the patch was removed at 7, I learnt to read at breakneck speed and developed a talent for all things academic. By 9, I was pushed up a class due to boredom, and by 10, my school arranged for a tutor to work with me on O-level maths papers. It was expected I would earn a scholarship to a grammar school, which I did. However, I also auditioned for a famous music school, as I'd shown a real flair for guitar, piano, and drums. I had developed perfect pitch and managed to complete all my piano grades in just two years. I suppose I was considered a child prodigy.

One thing to note: I found it much easier to express my emotions through the keys of a piano than through words, which pointed to my struggles with alexithymia.

At around 14, my grades began to slip as my concentration failed. I was marked down repeatedly for spelling mistakes, and in one exam, I lost full marks because

I forgot to write my name at the top. They only recognised my work because of my terrible handwriting, which could take several forms over a single page. The ADHD was really kicking in by this point.

I was highly strung, hyperactive, and habitually bullied throughout most of my childhood and into my early 20s.

During all this time, I never would have considered myself autistic or ADHD. Much of the negativity I experienced in my 20s and beyond, I attributed to trauma and the stress of boarding school and bullying. It was only in my mid-40s, when my depression and anxiety cycles became more frequent and extreme, that I finally reached out to a charity. They offered me support and helped me identify my autistic side.

The more I've learnt about my autistic identity, the kinder I can be to myself. And the kinder I am, the closer I feel to some form of contentment.

Now, I'm a music producer and composer, fortunate enough to have worked with some of the biggest artists in the world.

Life isn't so bad if you can stop for a minute and take a breath.

Joan Laplana

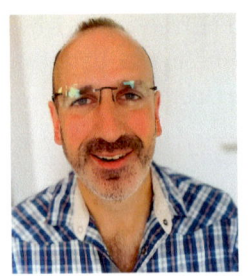

I am an autistic nurse originally from Barcelona, Spain. I spent my first 20 years living in a cosy 70-square-metre apartment in the vibrant Sagrada Familia neighbourhood, where my parents still reside. I was the youngest in the family and had a very happy childhood, but I always knew I was different. School was a struggle – I didn't fit in well and often found myself in detention, my mind constantly wandering while I longed for space to create and imagine. The rigid, repetitive learning style of my education felt suffocating. My English teacher once told my parents I was a waste of space and would never achieve anything. He even ranked students in order of ability, leaving me perpetually in the back row. Despite all of this, my parents supported me unconditionally, even taking me to a child psychologist when I was younger, though autism was never considered at the time.

Defying the odds, and with my parents' encouragement, I graduated as a nurse in 1997. For over 20 years now, I have lived in Sheffield, United Kingdom, where I have dedicated my career to transforming the healthcare system by championing equality, diversity, and inclusion at every level. My passion lies in empowering both frontline workers and patients to collaborate and lead change together.

Over the years, I've spearheaded national campaigns, lobbied for crucial reforms, and worked to inspire a healthcare system that truly values neurodiversity. Currently, I work with NHS England, where I support, mentor, and guide neurodivergent students to develop the skills and confidence they need to excel in the NHS. I also lead Choices College in South Yorkshire, a programme that defies national trends by achieving over 80% employment or apprenticeship outcomes for interns with learning disabilities or who are neurodivergent. This work not only transforms lives but also shifts workplace perceptions about neurodiversity and learning disabilities. In 2023, Choices College was recognised with the prestigious National Association for Special Educational Needs award for Best Specialist Provision of the Year – an achievement I'm incredibly proud of.

In addition to my work with the NHS and Choices College, I founded the Neurodiverse Nurses UK network, a platform that supports nurses with neurodivergent profiles, offering resources, education, and pastoral care. I'm also a mental health ambassador, leading initiatives like the Shiny Mind App and Doctors in Distress webinars to improve mental health support for healthcare professionals.

Beyond healthcare, I'm dedicated to raising understanding about diversity and inclusion across all sectors. In 2023, I was honoured to be included in the Global Health Excellence List by Zenith Global Health and the Diversity Power List 2023/24 as one of the UK's 50 most influential champions of inclusion.

My journey from a young boy in Barcelona who struggled to fit into the mould of traditional education to becoming a nurse, advocate, and leader in the UK's healthcare sector is a testament to the power of resilience and support. For me, anything is possible with the right mindset and backing, and I hope my work inspires others to break down barriers, create opportunities, and reimagine what's possible. You can learn more about me and my journey at www.RoaringNurse.com

Hazel Lim

I'm Hazel Lim, an autism advocate and proud founder of Chinese Autism CIC. I was born in Malaysia and moved to London in 2004 and work as an interpreter. I have three children, and my journey into autism advocacy began when my eldest son was five years old. I noticed he interacted and responded differently compared to his peers, though I couldn't quite pinpoint why.

I raised my concerns with his teachers, who suggested he might be neurodivergent and referred him for an assessment. However, with a waiting list of over two years, we were left without a diagnosis or the support we desperately needed. Determined to help my son, I began researching autism myself. But when I turned to friends and family for support, I was met with silence. While they had heard of autism, they didn't understand it or felt too uncomfortable to engage.

Feeling isolated, I knew I had to find my own way. In 2015, I gave up my career and moved my family to Swansea, Wales, to pursue an MSc in autism and related conditions at Swansea University. My studies deepened my understanding of autism and revealed the unique challenges faced by the Chinese community regarding stigma and misunderstanding. I decided to act.

In 2016, I founded the Chinese Autism Support Group to support Chinese families navigating autism. Then, in 2019, I produced the first bilingual English and Chinese autism booklet in the UK. This resource addressed the cultural barriers many families face and offered professionals insight into the challenges within our community. It's been widely used in Wales and internationally, and in 2021, I was honoured with a Prime Minister's Point of Light award for my work.

Over the years, I've been blessed to receive recognition through awards like Womenspire's Champion of Champions and UK Chinese Woman of the Year in volunteering. These accolades mean so much, but my true reward comes from seeing the positive impact on families and communities.

The road hasn't been easy. I've faced cultural stigma, deeply rooted misconceptions, and limited resources. Yet my desire to ensure no family suffers in silence keeps me going. In 2021, I founded Chinese Autism CIC to provide nationwide support and empower Chinese families with knowledge and guidance. Our mission is to transform stigma into strength by addressing prejudice, fostering inclusion, and creating a more compassionate society.

My own journey has also been one of discovery. In 2016, I was diagnosed as ADHD, and in 2022, as autism. Embracing my neurodivergence has been transformative. It's not just about understanding myself better; it's about celebrating the unique strengths it brings. My hyperfocus, attention to detail, and intuitive understanding of others have become my superpowers. These traits have fuelled my creativity, deepened my connections, and enriched my work.

As for my eldest son, he continues to face challenges as an autistic young man navigating a world designed for neurotypicals. Yet, he's thriving academically and is set to complete his A-levels this year with outstanding results. Cambridge University has already taken notice, offering him a place should he choose to go. His resilience inspires me every day.

Kosjenka Petek

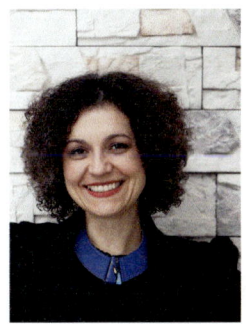

I'm Kosjenka Petek, an autistic teacher from Zagreb, Croatia. I'm a mother to one autistic teen and two service dogs, Bobby McGhee, a zen goldie, and Zoe Yvette, a feisty corgi.

As a teacher and teacher trainer, I love helping other educators grow their skills, especially in ways that make learning more inclusive and accessible for all students. My passion is making the world fairer for autistic kids and other marginalized groups.

I co-own and run Wisdom Tree edu center, and I love helping other educators grow their skills, especially in ways that make learning more inclusive and accessible for all students.

I'm also a proud self-advocate and volunteer with ASK, an autistic advocacy group in Croatia. As ASK's programme director, I work on designing and executing projects that promote inclusivity and equality, striving to establish spaces where everyone, regardless of their differences, feels valued, accepted, and loved for who they are. For example, in collaboration with my colleague, Eva Pavić, I conceptualised and now facilitate workshops called "Seeing Language." These workshops emphasise the human and educational rights of non-speaking and neurodivergent individuals, universal design in teaching, and the application of augmentative and alternative communication (AAC).

My intensive interests are participatory research, exploring the subject of alternative schools, and geeking out over *Doctor Who*. My autistic glimmers are reading, plant watching, cooking, finding joy in music, and all the little things that carry beauty and joy.

You can find out more about the work I do here: udrugaask.hr and wisdomtreecenter.com

Lyric Rivera

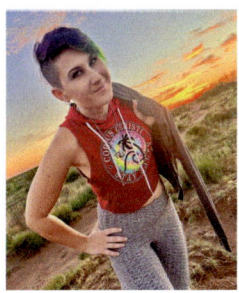

I'm Lyric Rivera, more widely known by my pseudonym, NeuroDivergent Rebel. I'm originally from Texas in the United States. While we're currently back in Texas, my partner and I recently returned from a two-year trip through the southwestern part of the country (mostly Colorado and New Mexico) in an RV with our dogs and hope to get back on the road before too long.

I am a multiply neurodivergent advocate, blogger, and best-selling author of the business ethics book *Workplace NeuroDiversity Rising*.

I spend most of my time educating about and advocating on behalf of neurodivergent people. However, I didn't know I was autistic (or even neurodivergent) for the first 29 years of my life – which had a profound impact on me.

My life before my autism discovery was one of suffering in silence, stuck in a world that didn't understand me.

People misunderstood me. Similarly, before learning the truth about my brain, I was unable to understand myself (because I thought I was something I was not – neurotypical).

I was neurodivergent, but I didn't know it yet, leaving me trapped in a cycle of self-doubt and confusion (trying to fit into a society that saw me as broken or wrong, punishing, scolding, mocking, and even physically harming me when I expressed neurodivergent traits).

Not knowing this truth for the first part of my life had devastating impacts on me. Before I knew the truth, I was constantly comparing myself to, and holding myself to, neurotypical standards.

I was also continually burning out and making myself physically and mentally ill.

Ever since learning I was autistic at the age of 29, I have been on a journey of healing and have been sharing that journey with the world via my blog.

I've dedicated my life to promoting acceptance, understanding, and inclusivity for autistic and other neurodivergent people worldwide.

Through my blog, *NeuroDivergent Rebel*, I share my experiences, insights, and perspectives on autism, neurodiversity, and social justice.

My writing is authentic, sometimes humorous, and unapologetically honest.

I'm passionate about challenging harmful stereotypes and stigmatizing narratives about neurodiversity and highlighting the strengths, creativity, contributions, and unique struggles of neurodivergent People.

By sharing my own deeply personal experiences with masking, meltdowns, societal expectations, and more, I aim to humanize and build a better global understanding of autistic and other neurodivergent people, helping our allies to develop a better sense of empathy and understanding for those of us whose minds work differently.

My work has inspired countless people to embrace their own neurodivergent brains and encouraged them to advocate for themselves and others.

Through my unwavering dedication and unapologetic voice, I aim to create a space where neurodivergent people are valued, respected, and empowered to be their authentic selves.

It is an honor to have my story used as an empowerment tool for future generations of neurodivergent people as they embark on their own self-discovery journeys.

I can be on my blog NeuroDivergentRebel.com or NeuroDivergentConsulting.org for organizations wanting help with their own neuro-inclusion efforts.

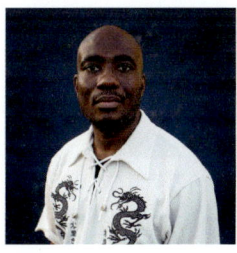

William Vanderpuye

I'm William Vanderpuye, a social worker with extensive experience in mental health and social care, currently working in the learning disabilities team for the London Borough of Sutton. My career has spanned several boroughs of London, from children's social care to adult mental health within the NHS.

Born in The Hague, Netherlands, to diplomat parents, my early life was shaped by travel, exposure to diverse cultures, and a love for languages. I grew up in France and Ghana, experiencing different but challenging forms of social exclusion. In France, I faced racial bullying but found acceptance in a small group of friends who taught me how to interact socially. Ghana, however, presented a different kind of challenge, where stigma against neurodivergence and disability was deeply entrenched. These experiences shaped my later passion for advocating for inclusion and acceptance.

My personal journey with autism began when I met an undiagnosed autistic student while I was teaching in a secondary school. This experience led me to reflect on my own experiences and realise I was autistic too. After my diagnosis in the UK, I became an advocate for neurodiversity, raising awareness of autism and fighting stigma, especially within Black communities. While some people embraced my diagnosis, others rejected it, perpetuating harmful myths about autism. This strengthened my resolve to challenge stereotypes and promote acceptance.

In July 2020, I joined the board of directors at Autistic Inclusive Meets (AIM), a grassroots organisation dedicated to creating opportunities for autistic individuals and their families. I also co-lead a growing social media group that provides support and encourages positive autistic identity. Through these platforms, I work to amplify autistic voices and challenge stigma.

Education has been central to my personal and professional journey. I hold a bachelor of arts in French and political science from the University of Ghana, an early years teacher status (EYTS) from Canterbury Christ Church University, a master of arts in early childhood studies from London Metropolitan University, and a master of arts in social work from Goldsmiths, University of London. These qualifications, combined with my lived experience, inform my approach to social work and advocacy.

Outside of work, I enjoy reading, playing the guitar, and singing. I have a keen interest in animals, from dogs and horses to snakes, ferrets, and tarantulas – I even ran a YouTube channel about my eight tarantulas at one point. I love spending time with my family – my wife, Afiba, who is a civil engineer, and our three daughters. Together, we blend our cultural heritage with our shared values, creating a home that celebrates diversity and inclusion.

Understanding the seven thematic categories

Each entry in this encyclopaedia is visually mapped against seven thematic categories, each represented by a unique symbol. These categories serve as navigational guides, grouping related terms and concepts, with the aim of enhancing the accessibility of this resource. The goal is to help readers navigate interconnected material more easily and locate information that is immediately meaningful to them. For example, someone interested in neurodivergent mental health can look for the relevant category symbol to quickly find all concepts directly and indirectly related to mental health. These symbols act as visual markers, making it easy to identify and explore entries belonging to a specific category at a glance.

These thematic categories are as follows:

🗨 Neurodivergent identities, states, and models

This category focuses on the broad spectrum of neurodivergent experiences, covering identities, neurotypes, and conceptual frameworks. Entries here introduce various neurological phenomena, characteristics, and ways of perceiving the world. The terms provide foundational knowledge that allows readers to appreciate the richness and complexity within the neurodivergent landscape.

🌿 Emotional and mental health and well-being

This category helps readers gain insight into the emotional landscape of neurodivergence, with the spotlight on the feelings, moods, and emotional states that influence the day-to-day lives of neurodivergent individuals.

👥 Social interaction, communication, and relationships

Neurodivergent individuals often communicate and relate to others in ways that differ from neurotypical people. This category delves into these differences, including the nuances of interactional styles and social engagement.

⚖ Advocacy, rights, and community dynamics

Neurodiversity is not only about individual experiences but also about collective action, societal frameworks, and the pursuit of justice. Terms in this category reflect this and, as such, include legal framework, key policies, and advocacy-related efforts to create a fairer world for neurodivergent individuals.

🛡 Support and therapy

This category groups terms related to supportive and therapeutic approaches, tools, and strategies designed to support neurodivergent needs. Whether describing assistive technology, sensory-friendly strategies, or therapeutic modalities, entries marked with this category guide readers towards supportive, non-stigmatising practices that honour neurodivergent autonomy and well-being.

🏢 Education and professional contexts

This category includes terms related to inclusive teaching methods and other forms of professional best practices. It is therefore a category for helping professionals keep up-to-date with the latest understanding associated with workplace and employment-related issues and concepts.

🚫 Harmful, pathologising, and stigmatising concepts and practices

This category encompasses so-called therapies, beliefs, policies, concepts, or frameworks that inherently cause harm, perpetuate stigma, or undermine the autonomy and well-being of neurodivergent people. Terms assigned to this category are not neutral or supportive; instead, they represent aspects of society or practices that neurodiversity advocates encourage people to be critical of, avoid, and, ultimately, dismantle.

Please note that each term may appear in one or more categories, reflecting the interconnectedness of these concepts.

A

Ableism

Ableism describes the discrimination and social prejudice against disabled people based on the belief that typical abilities are superior. It is a deeply problematic societal attitude that considers disabled people as needing to be 'fixed' or cured. Ableism often stems from a lack of understanding or appreciation for the diverse ways in which people experience the world, especially in the context of neurodivergence. It manifests in various forms, including the underestimation of the capabilities of disabled individuals and the systemic barriers that prevent full participation in society. For example, an employer might assume that an autistic person is less competent and therefore not hire them, or a public space may lack necessary accessibility features, excluding those with mobility impairments. Ableism can also lead to 'internalised ableism,' where disabled individuals believe the negative stereotypes and misconceptions about their own identities. This internalisation is extremely harmful to one's mental health, leading to feelings of worthlessness and self-doubt.

IN MY OWN WORDS: JOAN LAPLANA

Working in the wrong environment without the right support can be soul destroying. My story is a clear example. I am very creative and always had 100s of ideas, most of them useless but occasionally one of them is brilliant. But, unfortunately, at the beginning of my career I felt constricted by the hierarchical system, and I couldn't be myself or express my ideas properly. Every time that I tried to be myself it ended in disaster. I was told on many occasions that I was over-sensitive, aggressive, that I needed to stop challenging my managers and do as they tell me. I was getting in trouble at work on a regular basis.

This criticism was a manifestation of ableism, as my neurodivergent way of processing and expressing ideas was not appreciated or understood.

After being dismissed for the first time, I tried to fit and hide my personality. At that time, my family begging me to try to comply. I started to mask to be able to survive in a neurotypical world. Masking was my way of responding to ableism that I felt, but I became frustrated. After a while I began to experience negative feeling towards myself and work. I went home at the end of every shift demoralised, deflated and sad. My nursing career began to drift, I felt emotionally drained, and I even started to develop negative attitudes towards patients and coworkers, and a growing devaluation of my own competence. This internalised ableism led to a growing devaluation of my own competence, negatively impacting my care for patients and relationships with coworkers.

Despite my efforts to conform, I still ended up facing another 'fitness to practice' panel. This time my manager told me that I was not fit to be a nurse. I was devastated but looking at it in hindsight she was probably right. After more than 10 years of nursing in May 2012 decided that nursing was not for me anymore.

For the first time on my life, I was unemployed and claiming benefits. I felt useless and for the first time in my life suicide crossed my mind, but I wasn't brave enough. I nearly packed my bags and went back to Spain but somehow I didn't give up and after 4 months I decided to apply for a job as a community nurse. My manager and the whole team were fantastic. I felt supported and valued and had an environment free from ableism where my neurodivergence was seen as an asset rather than a liability. For the first time in my life, I was smiling at work. Six years later in 2018 I was named 'Best Nurse of The Year.'

Absence seizures

Often referred to as 'blank stare syndrome,' absence seizures involve sudden, brief lapses in consciousness typically lasting a few seconds. They manifest as a sudden 'zoning out' where the individual becomes momentarily unresponsive, sometimes with slight body movements like eye blinking or head nodding. Unlike other types of seizures, absence seizures do not involve convulsions and are often mistaken for daydreaming, making them hard to spot. They can both trigger and be triggered by hyperventilation, creating a self-perpetuating cycle, with healthcare professionals often needing to use controlled hyperventilation during diagnostic evaluations to provoke and observe absence seizures to aid in obtaining an accurate diagnosis. Absence seizures often start in childhood and, as such, are frequently misinterpreted and stigmatised as inattentiveness or bad behaviour. However, individuals who experience this require sensitive understanding and support, not stigma or negative judgements.

Acceptance ⚖ 🔵

Acceptance, within the context of neurodiversity, is a fundamental concept advocating for the recognition, respect, and appreciation of neurological differences as natural and valuable aspects of human diversity. It is much more than mere tolerance or awareness and instead involves actively embracing and valuing neurodivergent people for who they authentically are, without attempting to change their inherent neurological identity to conform to neurotypical standards.

Access arrangements ⚖ 🔵 🏢

Access arrangements are adaptations and accommodations made in various settings, like educational institutions, workplaces, and public spaces, to support the unique needs of neurodivergent people. These arrangements should ensure that neurodivergent people have equal opportunities to participate, perform, and excel in environments typically structured for neurotypicals. They involve modifications or supports tailored to individual needs, such as providing quiet spaces, alternative communication methods, flexible scheduling, or sensory-friendly environments. Access arrangements are not merely about physical accessibility but also encompass understanding and adapting to the cognitive, sensory, and social needs of autistic people. Implementing these arrangements is a fundamental aspect of creating inclusive, respectful, and empathetic environments that recognise and value neurodivergence.

Accessibility ⚖ 🔵 🏢

Accessibility refers to the quality or characteristic of something that makes it possible to plan for, approach, enter, and use it for positive gain. This goes beyond physical access to include cognitive, sensory, communicative and cultural aspects, ensuring environments and services are accessible for neurodivergent people. It encompasses a wide range of considerations, such as providing information in formats that suit different communication styles and needs – this might mean using literal, direct language for autistic individuals, providing materials in Braille for those who are visually impaired, offering sign language interpretation for Deaf individuals, providing assistive technology for non-speaking people, or offering information in multiple languages. Accessibility is vital in education, employment, healthcare, and public services, enabling neurodivergent people to participate fully and equitably in society.

ADHD 💬

ADHD, often termed 'attention deficit hyperactive disorder' in medical contexts, is increasingly recognised simply as attention differences, reflecting a shift away from pathologising language like 'deficit' and 'disorder.' ADHD is a form of neurodivergence that reflects unique ways of thinking, feeling, and experiencing the world. It is often characterised by cognitive and physical hyperactivity, impulsivity, and unique attention patterns. This can make ADHD individuals creative problem-solvers, passionate leaders, and dynamic contributors in their communities.

It is important to note that no two ADHD minds are the same and the expression of ADHD varies widely. For example, some may hyperfocus on tasks they love, achieving brilliance in bursts of energy, while others may juggle multiple ideas at once, thriving in high-stimulation environments.

Supporting ADHD individuals should not be about fixing or taming them but rather about creating a world that can accept, value, and leverage their unique abilities to make the world a brighter and more innovative place.

IN MY OWN WORDS: AGUSTINA CARDOSO

To me, ADHD feels like watching a fireworks show. Thoughts and ideas explode in a burst of colour and excitement, in unique and unpredictable ways. The initial rush of novelty is thrilling, a chaos of possibilities; you don't know where or when the next one is going to be and, for a moment, you can't look away. But as the show continues, it becomes overwhelming – too much brilliance, too much noise, too many fireworks bursting at the same time, and not enough capacity to pay attention to all of them. Suddenly, you become aware that you can't catch up with all of them, and the once dazzling display turns into an overload of sensory information to process.

Life is not a fireworks show, but every day we are flooded by sensory information that demands our attention, whether we consent to it or not. For ADHD brains, this sensory onslaught is amplified. It's like every notification, every conversation, every flickering light competes for centre stage, turning the world into a relentless fireworks display.

ADHD brains are creative, innovative, and driven. When we focus on something we like, we enter a state of hyperfocus, and the possibilities to build something feel limitless. But when we force our brains to focus on what it doesn't want, we struggle to manage the relentless flood of thoughts and tasks. The internal struggle to focus gets externalised, and suddenly we can't sit still – we are fidgeting, tapping, and pacing. Time and energy management dissolve – we miss deadlines, forget tasks, and exhaust ourselves in the process.

The idea of understanding ADHD as a difference in attention regulation feels the most accurate for me, as it precisely illustrates the struggle many of us face daily. When deadlines feel like insurmountable walls, when an office becomes a sensory hell, when your to-do list piles up into metres and metres of undone tasks, it's easy to feel broken. It's not about a deficit in attention skills but a deficit in the current system that expects all brains to function the same.

Adjustments vs accommodations ⚖️

'Adjustments' and 'accommodations' are terms often used interchangeably in the context of creating inclusive environments for neurodivergent individuals. However, they can carry slightly different connotations.

Adjustments refer to changes made to existing structures, practices, or policies to better enable neurodivergent individuals to participate fully in various settings like workplaces, schools, or public areas. This might include altering communication methods, providing flexible work or study schedules, or modifying assessment methods. The emphasis here is on modifying existing frameworks to become more inclusive.

Accommodations, however, refer to the provision of additional services, support, or equipment to assist neurodivergent individuals that were not originally present in the environment. This could, for example, encompass providing sensory-friendly environments, assistive technology, or one to one support.

Advocacy ⚖️ 🛡️

Advocacy, within the realm of neurodiversity, involves actively supporting and promoting the interests and rights of neurodivergent people who are often marginalised or misunderstood in society. This involves challenging stereotypes, confronting discriminatory practices, and working towards systemic change in areas like education, employment, health and social care, and social policy. It also includes personal advocacy, where individuals advocate for their own needs.

Effective advocacy requires empathy, understanding, and a deep respect for the neurodivergent experience. Advocates must listen to and amplify the voices of neurodivergent individuals, promote their autonomy, and ensure that they have the same opportunities to thrive as their neurotypical peers.

IN MY OWN WORDS: HAZEL LIM

In my role as a multilingual autism specialist in the UK, I have witnessed firsthand the significant challenges that Chinese immigrants face when dealing with neurodivergence. Many families struggle to comprehend and accept diagnoses due to cultural stigma and a lack of accessible information. This struggle is compounded by the complexity of navigating healthcare, education, and support systems, which can seem overwhelmingly complicated.

Chinese families frequently face additional barriers, including language difficulties and cultural stigma surrounding autism and neurodivergence. These barriers can make it exceptionally hard for them to articulate their needs and seek the support they require. The process of accepting a neurodivergent identity is often prolonged, exacerbated by an environment that may not be fully accepting or supportive.

To address these challenges, I have committed myself to advocating for Chinese neurodivergent individuals and their families. I serve on various boards, including national health boards, government neurodiversity advisory boards, and local parent carer groups. My goal is to ensure that the unique barriers faced by Chinese neurodivergent individuals are recognised and addressed.

A significant part of my advocacy involves raising awareness about the specific challenges these individuals face. Many service providers may not be aware of the cultural and linguistic barriers that Chinese families encounter. By highlighting these issues, I aim to create a more inclusive and understanding environment within healthcare and support services.

Advocacy is not always an easy task, and it is often not something I enjoy. However, I am deeply motivated by the knowledge that my efforts are helping to represent many unheard voices. These individuals, who might be suffering due to language barriers and cultural stigma, deserve to have their needs recognised and addressed.

One of the most rewarding aspects of my advocacy work has been seeing the gradual improvements in service provision. By collaborating with various boards and organisations, we have been able to implement changes that make services more accessible and inclusive. This includes providing 'non-stigmatised' translated materials, cultural competency training for service providers, and establishing support networks that are sensitive to the cultural needs of Chinese families.

Through these efforts, I have seen families become more empowered to seek the support they need. Parents who once felt isolated and overwhelmed now have the resources and understanding to advocate for their children effectively, and acceptance has been fostering. Children who were once marginalised are now receiving more of the support and acceptance they need to thrive.

Despite the challenges, my advocacy work is driven by a deep commitment to creating a more inclusive society. Every time I speak out, I remind myself that I am giving a voice to those who may not be able to speak for themselves. This responsibility is both a privilege and a driving force behind my continued efforts.

In conclusion, advocacy for Chinese neurodivergent individuals is about much more than raising awareness. It is about creating tangible changes that improve lives. It is about breaking down barriers and fostering an environment where all individuals, regardless of their cultural background or neurodivergent status, can thrive. Through my work, I hope to continue making a positive impact and ensuring that every voice is heard and valued.

Affective empathy

Affective empathy is the emotional response that occurs when one feels or mirrors the emotions of others. It is an automatic, often unconscious, reaction to another's emotional state and leads to a shared emotional experience. It can also include empathising deeply with animals, fictional characters, and objects. For autistic people, affective empathy can manifest intensely and unpredictably, sometimes causing overwhelming emotional responses that are difficult to manage or express, particularly in environments that lack sensory accommodations or understanding. They might also struggle to express it in ways that align with neurotypical social norms, leading to misconceptions and negative judgement, including false assertion that autistic people lack empathy altogether. However, in reality, these differences highlight the 'double empathy problem,' which reflects the mutual misunderstandings between autistic and non-autistic individuals.

Affiliate stigma

Affiliate stigma emerges when the stigma associated with neurodivergence is internalised by those closely linked to neurodivergent individuals, such as parents, caregivers, other family members. This internalisation leads these 'affiliates' to experience self-stigma, even if they are not neurodivergent themselves.

Affiliate stigma arises from the existence of public stigma, which creates the social conditions necessary for its development. Eliminating public stigma is therefore a critical step in preventing affiliate stigma and other forms of secondary stigma, such as internalised stigma and internalised ableism. In addition, empowering individuals to resist and reject stigma can help reduce its internalisation and harmful effects.

Addressing affiliate stigma is essential for safeguarding the mental health of those within a neurodivergent individual's support network, as it can profoundly affect their psychological well-being and the quality of care they provide.

Affinity cycle

The term 'affinity cycle' describes the strong attachments neurodivergent individuals, particularly autistic people, often form with specific affinities – deep interests or passions – that provide predictability, sensory regulation, and comfort in an often overwhelming world. These affinities might include certain foods, music, TV shows, or hobbies, and they offer a reliable source of control and relief amidst sensory and social unpredictability.

However, this state is not permanent; it can end suddenly, resulting in an intense and sometimes overwhelming aversion to the previously cherished stimulus. While this intolerance may appear puzzling to others, it is typically temporary, and a return to the initial preference may eventually follow. The sudden shift from preference to aversion may be linked to sensory saturation, wherein overstimulation overwhelms the sensory system or, perhaps, due to shifts in internal regulation needs, causing the brain to seek alternative sensory input.

Affinity therapy and passion-based therapies

These are therapeutic approaches that centre around the specific interests and passions of neurodivergent individuals to engage, support, and connect with them.

In affinity therapy, the therapist actively incorporates the individual's specific interests into the therapy sessions in a structured way. This can create a more engaging and comfortable environment for the autistic individual, facilitating better communication, learning, and social interaction. For example, if an autistic person is passionate about gardening, the therapist might use gardening-related scenarios to navigate social interactions and boost self-efficacy.

Passion-based therapies, on the other hand, adopt a broader framework, using the individual's passions as a foundation to support well-being. This often involves engaging the person in activities or discussions related to their passions but are less focused on integrating these interests into the therapy process itself. For example, a person with a deep love for trains might be encouraged to pursue train-related projects to build confidence and develop practical skills.

Both approaches celebrate and validate the unique ways neurodivergent individuals experience the world, offering a respectful, person-centred alternative to traditional, often pathologising therapies.

Alexithymia

Also sometimes referred to as 'emotional blindness,' alexithymia is commonly experienced within the autistic and broader neurodivergent community. It involves difficulty in identifying, describing, and expressing one's own emotions. This can lead to misunderstandings in social interactions, as emotional expressions might not align with typical expectations.

Alexithymia does not mean a lack of emotion, nor does it mean that an individual cannot experience empathy or even hyperempathy. In fact, some people with alexithymia may find themselves profoundly affected by others' emotions without being able to clearly understand or express their own.

Alexithymia adds another layer of complexity to the already diverse ways neurodivergent people experience and interact with the world. Supporting alexithymia involves creating environments where various ways of experiencing and expressing emotions are accepted and where individuals are given the space and tools to understand and articulate their feelings in their own time and manner, and without judgement.

IN MY OWN WORDS: JORIS FOUET

Imagine you're plate-spinning. Constantly going from one plate to another, keeping everything turning, regulating discreetly, here and there, every now and then, so the whole thing looks stable from the outside.

It's not stable. It'll collapse as soon as you stop maintaining it. And hell, you might break a plate along the way and keep going. But with a little practice, it seems possible.

Alexithymia is doing the same thing, but blindfolded.

You can hear the plates, you can tap to accelerate them, you know when one falls down. But how fast is it spinning? The only way to know is by touching a plate and sensing how it slows down or accelerates.

For example, I'll be working on something and notice that my palms are sweating and my heart is racing. I notice it because I do conscious checks on vitals whenever I'm not sure.

So next up, likely causes: I haven't been running, so it's probably something going on around me.

Maybe I just don't like this place. I'll wrap up what I have to do and get out of here. So I double down.

Next day, I'll be talking to someone who was working on the same thing, and they'll tell me it was so frustrating they had to take breaks regularly.

We both needed a break. The thought just didn't occur to me. Quite the opposite, I would have never guessed that it was the work. Because usually, it's the environment.

I cannot, for the life of me, tell the difference between frustration and exhaustion. I can analyse how intense it is at any given time; I've learned to watch out for warning signs, but aside from strong and weak, I don't have any useful categories. I can't really say even if it's good or bad. I can only tell you how much it overwhelms my purely analytical approach.

All Age Autism Guidance

The All Age Autism Guidance by NHS England outlines a comprehensive, evidence-based framework for autism assessments across all ages. Prioritising accessibility and respect for diverse needs, it defines a five-stage pathway covering identification, referral, assessment, and pre- and post-assessment support. The guidance emphasises personalised care, informed consent, and approaches like social prescribing and shared decision-making, ensuring support aligns with individual needs. By addressing the entire assessment process, it aims to provide a holistic and inclusive approach to autism diagnosis and care.

Allistic

Allistic is a non-pathologising term used to describe individuals who are not autistic. The term highlights the diversity of neurological experiences rather than framing autism as a deviation from a so-called 'norm.' It is derived from the Greek root *allos*, meaning 'other.'

By recognising allistic individuals as simply one of many neurotypes, the use of 'allistic' helps dismantle the autistic/non-autistic binary. It challenges the assumption that being non-autistic equates to a 'normal' or 'standard' neurological state and instead reframes all neurotypes as equally valid expressions of human diversity.

Allyship

Allyship is the active, consistent, and arduous practice of using privilege to support, uplift, and advocate for others. For neurodivergent people, effective allyship requires a long-term commitment to learning about the experiences and challenges they face, listening to their voices, and respecting their autonomy and perspectives. It also involves actively challenging ableist attitudes and practices in various environments, including the workplace, educational settings, and social interactions. Allies play a crucial role in promoting acceptance, creating inclusive spaces, and supporting policies and practices that respect and celebrate neurological differences.

Aloneness

Aloneness is the experience or preference for solitude often observed among autistic individuals. It can be distinguished from loneliness, which, instead, implies a lack of desired social interaction. Aloneness, on the contrary, reflects a comfortable state where an autistic person may find solace, rejuvenation, or enjoyment in being alone. It is a state where they can engage deeply with personal interests, process thoughts and experiences, or simply enjoy a sensory environment tailored to their preferences. This term is critical in understanding that solitude for autistic individuals is not necessarily indicative of social deficits or isolation but rather a self-determined and fulfilling aspect of their neurology.

Alternative assessment methods

Unlike traditional methods, which focus on standardised testing and normative performance metrics, alternative assessment methods aim to value and connect with the diverse ways in which neurodivergent individuals process information, learn, and express their knowledge and skills, thus creating an inclusive and equitable assessment landscape. These methods might include flexible testing environments, varied communication options (like oral presentations or visual projects), and assessments focusing on problem-solving and creativity rather than rote memorisation. This approach recognises and nurtures the strengths inherent in neurodivergence rather than penalising individuals for not fitting into a conventional educational or evaluative mould.

Angelman syndrome 🗨

Angelman syndrome is genetic condition, which occurs in approximately 1 in 15,000 live births, is primarily caused by a change or deletion on chromosome 15 and often associated with a missing or dysfunctional UBE3A gene inherited from the mother.

Angelman syndrome individuals often embody a unique and joyful presence, known for their frequent laughter, expressive happiness, and enthusiasm. They may also experience developmental delays, balance and coordination challenges, epilepsy, disrupted sleep, and complex communication needs. Despite limited speaking communication, most can understand language and use non-speaking methods to express themselves.

Animal-assisted therapy 🛡

The term 'animal-assisted therapy' (AAT) refers to the therapeutic process of incorporating trained animals and their handlers to collaborate with other professionals to support individuals in achieving specific physical, emotional, social, or cognitive goals. It is often incorporated in settings such as hospitals, schools, or care homes. The sessions may involve different activities such as grooming, petting, or walking the animal, depending on the individual's needs and the type of animal used.

For autistic people, AAT can offer benefits such as sensory regulation or low-demand social interaction, yet its implementation must centre the individual's preferences and comfort. Forced engagement, reliance on animal interaction to replace genuine human acceptance, or a lack of understanding of sensory needs can risk causing harm. Ethical considerations, particularly around the welfare of the animals involved, must also be prioritised to ensure a balanced and respectful approach. AAT should be one tool among many, not a panacea.

Anomic aphasia 🗨

Anomic aphasia, or nominal aphasia, is a neurological condition where individuals struggle to recall names of objects, people, or concepts, despite otherwise fluent speech and intact comprehension. It often stems from neurological injuries or conditions like strokes or degenerative diseases affecting language-related areas of the brain. These word-finding challenges can lead to frustration and social anxiety, particularly in conversational settings.

For neurodivergent individuals with anomic aphasia, the condition may intersect with existing communication differences, making inclusive strategies even more critical. For example, an autistic individual with anomic aphasia might find the dual challenges of word-finding and navigating neurotypical social norms overwhelming, especially in high-pressure environments like group discussions. Support can include augmentative and alternative communication tools, visual aids, contextual cues, and encouraging multimodal expression, such as gestures or writing. Creating patient, supportive environments and training communication partners to use empathetic techniques can help reduce stress and empower individuals to express themselves fully and authentically.

Anthropomorphising

Anthropomorphising is the act of attributing human traits, feelings, or intentions to non-human entities like animals, robots, objects, or abstract concepts. It is a natural human behaviour that helps people connect with and relate to the world. For many neurodivergent individuals, anthropomorphising can enable the expression of emotions and manage anxiety in a safe, low-demand and controllable way.

Unfortunately, however, anthropomorphising is often subject to stigma and misunderstanding, particularly when practised by neurodivergent individuals. For example, when an autistic person confides in a stuffed animal, it may be dismissed as 'childish' or misinterpreted as a sign of low intelligence. In contrast, neurotypicals are frequently praised for anthropomorphising in ways deemed creative or charming – such as naming their car, assigning personalities to pets, or creating whimsical stories about inanimate objects. These double standards highlight a broader societal bias that undervalues autistic ways of interacting with the world, framing them as deficits rather than meaningful expressions of individuality.

Anxiety

Anxiety is a significant and pervasive experience for neurodivergent individuals, particularly autistic people, and is one of the most crucial factors influencing their ability to cope and thrive in life. However, it is also one of the most vulnerable aspects, often undermined by many factors including stigma, ableism, and the daily struggles of living in a world designed for non-autistic individuals. A strong need for predictability and routine further amplifies this, as unexpected changes can trigger intense anxiety.

The effort to 'mask' autistic traits to blend into non-autistic environments is both a cause and consequence of anxiety, creating a vicious cycle. Those who experience heightened anxiety are more likely to mask to avoid judgement or discomfort, but this masking intensifies anxiety further, leading to exhaustion and emotional burnout. Conversely, individuals with lower anxiety levels are more likely to feel safe being their authentic selves, reducing the need for masking and improving mental well-being.

Despite its profound impact, anxiety is often treated superficially. Professionals too often recommend medication as a first-line solution without addressing the environmental and social factors that contribute to anxiety or equipping individuals with strategies to manage it. While medication can be beneficial in some cases, recognising and addressing these root causes are essential.

Aphantasia

Aphantasia is a neurological variation in which an individual has non-typical or limited ability to create mental imagery. This can make it difficult to visualise faces, scenes from books, or past experiences, impacting memory, daydreaming, and creative engagement. Despite this, it does not limit imagination or creativity, as many with aphantasia find alternative ways to process and express ideas. Interestingly, most can still experience vivid visual dreams, showing that while conscious visualisation is affected, the brain retains its capacity for involuntary imagery during sleep.

Aphantasia can also extend beyond visuals, affecting the ability to imagine sounds, tastes, or sensations. Many people only recognise they have aphantasia in adulthood, when they realise their experience differs from others'. Understanding aphantasia challenges the assumption that everyone can create mental images and broadens our appreciation of the many ways people think, process, and interact with the world.

Aphasia

Aphasia is a neurological phenomenon that affects a person's ability to comprehend, speak, read, or write. It is often misunderstood as simply a speech impairment, but it involves broader challenges with processing and producing language, usually due to brain injuries like strokes. The experience of aphasia varies widely – some people might struggle to find specific words, while others face greater difficulty forming or understanding sentences.

Importantly, aphasia does not reflect reduced intelligence; it is a difference in accessing language, not in the capacity to think or understand. Supporting someone with aphasia requires patience, respect, and adaptability, tailoring communication to their needs. This might mean using gestures, visual aids, or assistive technologies to ensure conversations remain inclusive and empowering.

Appeals

Appeals play a vital role in challenging decisions made by educational or healthcare institutions, especially when those decisions fail to meet the needs or respect the rights of neurodivergent individuals. Families, carers, advocates, or neurodivergent people themselves often turn to the appeals process when they disagree with assessments, support plans, or the provision of services. These appeals are essential to ensure that individual needs are properly recognised and met.

The process of appealing is not just about correcting errors – it is about upholding the legal rights of neurodivergent individuals and ensuring that institutions provide the support they need to succeed. While stressful and time-consuming, appeals are a powerful way to safeguard agency, amplify voices, and reinforce the principle that every neurodivergent person deserves to thrive in environments designed with their strengths and challenges in mind.

Applied behavioural analysis

Applied behavioural analysis (ABA) is a behavioural therapy approach that focuses on modifying behaviours through reinforcement techniques. While widely used, it has faced significant criticism for prioritising the alteration of natural autistic behaviours to fit neurotypical norms. This focus can disregard an individual's authentic self, often leading to internalised ableism, psychological distress, and long-term harm.

Rather than aiming to 'correct' intrinsic behaviours, support should prioritise acceptance, understanding and empowerment. Embracing neurodivergent ways of being involves respecting each person's unique needs and experiences, valuing them as they are rather than trying to change them. This shift away from behaviour modification affirms the richness of neurodivergent perspectives and enables a society that celebrates neurodivergence as a vital and enriching part of humanity.

Apraxia

Apraxia is a neurological phenomenon that affects an individual's ability to carry out planned movements or gestures, even when they know what they want to do and have the physical ability to do it. This disruption in motor planning can make it difficult to turn thoughts into purposeful actions. It can manifest as limb apraxia, involving challenges with intentional arm or leg movements, or verbal apraxia (apraxia of speech), which affects speech articulation.

For autistic individuals, apraxia can further complicate communication and daily tasks. Interestingly, automatic movements, like waving goodbye, often remain intact, while the same actions become difficult when consciously attempted.

Support strategies include breaking tasks into smaller steps, using visual aids, maintaining consistent routines, and allowing extra processing time. Access to occupational or speech therapy can also help individuals build confidence and reduce stress.

Art-based therapy

Art-based therapies use creative activities like drawing, painting, sculpture, or digital art as tools for self-expression and communication. This approach values the unique ways neurodivergent individuals perceive and interact with the world, providing an inclusive and supportive therapeutic medium.

Art-based therapy is especially valuable for those who find speaking-based communication challenging. It allows individuals to process emotions, experiences, and ideas in ways that feel natural and accessible, enabling self-awareness, emotional regulation, and coping skills while promoting a sense of accomplishment and personal growth.

In a neurodivergent-affirming context, art-based therapies prioritise choice, autonomy, and creativity, encouraging exploration without imposing neurotypical standards. This approach not only supports individual well-being but also celebrates neurodivergent ways of being, contributing to a more inclusive and compassionate society.

Articulation difficulties

Articulation difficulties refers to challenges some neurodivergent people face in producing clear or conventional speech sounds. Traditionally seen as an issue requiring 'correction,' it is essential to support and value different speech styles as valid forms of expression so they are accepted and supported rather than stigmatised.

For example, an autistic individual may have difficulty pronouncing certain sounds or structuring speech in ways that align with neurotypical expectations. Instead of correcting or dismissing their speech, a respectful and inclusive approach might involve giving them ample time to express themselves, using visual aids to supplement communication, or engaging in active listening to validate their effort and perspective. Speech and language therapists trained in neurodivergent-affirming practices can also provide support focused on enhancing clarity and confidence without pressuring individuals to conform to rigid norms.

Artificial intelligence and large language models

Artificial intelligence (AI) and large language models (LLMs) are increasingly influential in the realm of technology and communication, with profound implications for the neurodivergent community.

AI refers to the development of computer systems capable of learning, decision-making, problem-solving, and more. LLMs, a subset of AI, are advanced algorithms trained to understand and generate human-like text. They can perform a variety of language-related tasks, such as translation, summarisation, and answering questions.

For the neurodivergent community, AI and LLMs offer both opportunities and challenges. On one hand, they can provide assistive tools that support communication and learning. For example, AI-powered apps can assist individuals in interpreting emotions or managing daily tasks. On the other hand, there are concerns about AI and LLMs perpetuating biases or misunderstanding neurodivergent modes of communication.

As AI and LLMs continue to evolve, it is essential to involve neurodivergent voices in their development to ensure these technologies are inclusive, accessible, and respectful of neurodiversity. This ensures that the benefits of AI and LLMs can be fully realised by everyone, including those in the neurodivergent community.

IN MY OWN WORDS: JORIS FOUET

Learning a language is hard. It takes years for the best of us. It took decades for computers! But LLMs are here now. It's not exactly speech, but they can manipulate the language representation of an idea just as well as humans do.

How? Long story short: we mapped every single concept to every single word (and that's a very dense map), and then we can engineer sentences from there, by daisy-chaining those units of meaning. Which sounds exactly like the autistic language hypothesis. Makes you wonder who came up with it.

We have a joke in the software industry that society shouldn't have let autistic people design their interactions. Then again, we are the ones most likely to study them in depth.

That said, the LLM is not thinking: it'll never have an original idea, but given an idea, it can explain it in the perfect way for each and any audience. As such, it might be the bridge that connects us through the double-empathy problem; it can be the link that understands both neurotypical and neurodivergent ways of communicating. Maybe we can finally carry an idea from one brain to the next without distorting it at the interface.

Or maybe, on the contrary, since every language carries assumptions, boiling them all down to a single map will lose some valuable nuance.

Fun times.

For now, it certainly has become my go-to brainstormer. Whenever I have an interaction I don't understand, I'll run it through an LLM and I can analyse in excruciating detail what happened. I can ponder alternative interpretations. Compare them to expectations.

People tend to get annoyed pretty quickly when I ask them repeatedly what they mean. With an LLM, I can spar as much as I want, and more importantly, as much as I need. I can hone in on the meaning that matches most the corpus it learned from. I get to interrogate all the outputs of all the brains. Put it another way, I have access to what is neurologically typical.

#AskingAutistics

The hashtag '#AskingAutistics.' created by Lyric Rivera, represents a significant online movement that emerged on social media platforms to amplify and engage with the voices, experiences, and perspectives of autistic people. This cultural movement challenges traditional hierarchies of knowledge where neurotypical medical professionals and other external so-called experts dominate discussions about autism. Instead, this approach acknowledges autistic people as the most credible voices on their lives, needs, and identities. By using the hashtag, all individuals, including non-autistics, can respectfully tap into an array of insights directly from autistic voices. This ultimately enables inclusivity, shifts conversations away from ableist narratives, and helps build a richer societal understanding of autism and neurodivergence.

IN MY OWN WORDS: LYRIC RIVERA

As the originator of the #AskingAutistics hashtag I wanted to create a platform where Autistic People could share their experiences and perspectives without judgement or assumption.

It was also equally important to create a space where non-autistic people (or those who wonder if they MIGHT be Autistic) could engage with our community, asking whatever questions they could think of – because, at the time, no such resource was available (to my knowledge).

We had #ActuallyAutistic, but this hashtag is and always has been ONLY for Autistic People to use, so people who use it who are not Autistic are often ignored, scolded, or berated (because Autistic People don't have many spaces that are "just for us" or that only amplify our voices).

I believe that Autistic People are the best authorities on our own lives and experiences and that our voices should be centered on conversations about

Autism. However, without a bridge that allowed non-autistics (and suspected Autistics) into our world, a massive gap in understanding held us back. So, in 2016, I launched the hashtag on Twitter, hoping to build that "bridge," allowing a friendly curiosity to creep into our spaces through the hashtag #AskingAutistics.

I was tired of seeing non-autistic individuals dominate the conversation about Autism, often perpetuating harmful stereotypes and stigmatizing language. Still, I was also equally tired of witnessing Autistic People chasing potential allies (and undiagnosed Autistics) out of our community.

The response was overwhelming.

Autistic People, suspected Autistic People, and allies worldwide began using the hashtag to ask and answer questions and unite with others.

The hashtag became a safe space to connect, share, and support one another. It also became a resource for non-autistic individuals who wanted to learn about and understand Autism from our perspective.

Years later, the hashtag thrives, sparking conversations and connections that transcend borders and physical boundaries. It has become a symbol of Autistic empowerment and a reminder that our voices matter.

#AskingAutistics is a vital conversation starter in the online Autistic Community, empowering Autistic People to share our stories and assert our knowledge on Autism-related topics (because historically, we've been spoken over).

#AskingAutistics has also helped foster a sense of community and solidarity among Autistic People (who often face isolation). Through sharing our experiences and connecting with others who understand our struggles and triumphs, many of us have found validation, support, and (if we're lucky) a sense of community and belonging.

I am proud to have contributed to the creation of this hashtag and grateful to the countless individuals (both Autistic and non-autistic) who have contributed to its growth and success over the years by asking and answering questions.

As I look back on the journey of #AskingAutistics, I am reminded of the power of community and the importance of listening to and amplifying marginalized voices.

By using and engaging with this hashtag, we can work towards a more inclusive and accepting society where Autistic voices are placed front and center when discussing the Autistic Experience.

Asperger's

The term 'Asperger's,' once used to describe a specific manifestation of autism, is now widely seen as outdated and best replaced by the term 'autism.' Initially used to label a perceived subtype of autism characterised by traits like average or above-average intelligence and stronger language skills, the term has been criticised for reinforcing unhelpful and inaccurate stereotypes. It also introduced the problematic concept of 'high-functioning,' which creates a reductive and misleading hierarchy based on external functionality rather than acknowledging diverse and dynamic support needs.

The term's origin further adds to its controversy, as Hans Asperger, from whom it derives, was associated with Nazi eugenics programmes. Moving beyond these outdated and divisive labels allows for a more inclusive understanding of autism as a natural variation in human neurology.

Assistive technology

Assistive technology refers to devices or systems that support and empower neurodivergent people, particularly those who face challenges with communication, learning, and sensory processing. These tools range from common aids like noise-cancelling headphones, which help reduce sensory overload, to sophisticated communication devices and software tailored for those with speech and language differences. Such technology enables independence and self-expression, enabling individuals to participate more fully in education, employment, and social interactions while enriching their ability to engage in everyday life and access environments more effectively.

However, for these technologies to truly make a difference, their development and implementation must be shaped by the actual needs and preferences of neurodivergent people, ensuring the solutions are supportive, practical, and aligned with their lived experiences rather than conforming to neurotypical standards.

AuDHD

AuDHD is an informal term used to describe individuals who are both autistic and ADHD (attention deficit hyperactivity disorder), recognising the unique interplay of both neurodivergent identities. Autistic people may experience heightened sensory sensitivities, hyperfocus, hyperempathy, and difficulties with social communication, particularly when interacting with neurotypicals in environments that are not neurodivergent-affirming, while ADHD may bring characteristics such as hyperactivity, impulsivity, and differences in attention regulation. AuDHD acknowledges that these two neurotypes coexisting can create distinct patterns of behaviour and cognition needs that differ from those of people who are either solely autistic or solely ADHD. For instance, hyperfocus – often associated with autism – might blend with ADHD's attention differences, leading to a simultaneous deep engagement with some tasks and difficulty managing others.

Auditory processing disorder

Auditory processing disorder (APD) is recognised as a distinctive way in which some individuals interpret auditory information, diverging from typical auditory processing. APD is characterised by consistent challenges in the efficient and effective processing of sounds, including difficulties in distinguishing and interpreting speech in noisy environments. This divergence is not indicative of a deficit in hearing ability, per se, but rather in the brain's processing of auditory signals, particularly in the auditory pathways and centres of the brain.

The neurological processes involved in APD include auditory decoding (deciphering different sounds and speech elements), auditory figure-ground discrimination (focusing on important auditory information amidst background noise), auditory memory (short-term and working memory for sounds and language), and auditory integration (combining auditory information from both ears for coherent understanding). In APD, these processes may not function typically, leading to challenges such as difficulty following spoken instructions, understanding speech in noisy settings, or differentiating similar-sounding words.

Auditory sense

The auditory sense pertains to the ability to perceive and process sounds, encompassing not just the mechanical act of hearing but also the intricate neural processing of auditory information. This involves the transformation of sound waves into electrical signals by the inner ear, which the brain then interprets to make sense of language, music, and environmental sounds.

Yet, this sense is far more than a physiological function – it is a richly diverse neurological experience. For example, some autistic people may experience hyperacusis, where everyday sounds like the hum of a refrigerator or the rustle of paper feel unbearably loud or even painful, making environments that others find ordinary feel overwhelming. Conversely, others may have difficulty differentiating speech from background noise, such as in a crowded room, where every sound competes for attention, making it challenging to focus on conversations. These unique auditory experiences not only shape how autistic individuals perceive and interact with the world but also highlight the incredible variability and complexity of human sensory processing.

Augmentative and alternative communication 👥 🟦

Augmentative and alternative communication (AAC) refers to the methods and tools used to support or replace spoken language for individuals who face challenges in verbal communication. AAC encompasses a wide range of strategies, from non-technological approaches like sign language and picture boards to advanced technological solutions such as voice output communication aids. These tools and methods provide a voice to those whose verbal communication may be limited, facilitating their expression of thoughts, needs, and desires.

AAC is not merely a compensatory mechanism but an affirmation of the diverse ways in which individuals communicate and interact with the world. Recognising and incorporating AAC in educational, social, and professional settings is a critical step towards inclusivity, validating the unique communication styles of neurodivergent people.

Augmented reality 🟦 🏢

Augmented reality (AR) is a technology that overlays digital information onto the real world, often via smartphones or smart glasses, enhancing how users perceive their surroundings. By integrating virtual elements like images, sounds, or other sensory inputs with the environment in real time, AR opens up exciting possibilities for neurodivergent individuals.

For example, AR can create immersive, interactive learning environments tailored to unique sensory needs and learning styles, making educational content more engaging and accessible. It can also provide a calming, controlled space to help manage sensory overload or navigate challenging situations, offering significant potential for supporting mental health and well-being.

AuSocial 💬 👥

The term 'AuSocial,' a portmanteau of 'autistic' and 'social', represents a nuanced understanding of social interaction within the autistic community. Contrary to prevailing stereotypes that autistic people prefer isolation, 'AuSocial' acknowledges that autistic people often seek and value social connections, albeit in ways that differ from neurotypical norms. This concept challenges the misconception of autistic people as inherently antisocial or lacking in social skills. Instead, it emphasises that their social engagement, preferences, and methods of communication are distinctively shaped by their neurology. 'AuSocial' interactions may not conform to typical social expectations, such as eye contact or small talk, favouring more direct, honest, and deeply authentic communication styles that reflect their genuine social preferences.

Authentic self 💬 🌿

This refers to the practice of embracing and expressing one's true neurodivergent identity without feeling the need to mask or conform to societal expectations. For autistic people, it means living in a way that aligns with their natural communication, sensory, and emotional styles, rejecting pressures to adapt to neurotypical norms. The concept is rooted in the idea that neurodivergent identities are valid, valuable, and do not require suppression. Promoting the authentic self also challenges the stigma and negative assumptions surrounding neurodivergent people. This is why it is so important for creating environments where autistic people can feel safe and accepted as this encourages authenticity and mitigates the negative impacts of masking, such as anxiety or exhaustion.

Autie 💬

'Autie' is an affectionate, colloquial term embraced within the autistic community. It serves as both an identity label and a term of endearment among many autistic people. The term symbolises a positive shift away from pathologised, medicalised views of autism towards a more humanised and personal understanding of being autistic. It is part of a broader cultural movement that views autistic identity as a distinct and valued variation in human neurology, encouraging pride and acceptance instead of framing autism as a disorder or deficit.

IN MY OWN WORDS: GINNY GRANT

We began using 'Autie' in our home around the time of my formal identification as Autistic. Just as in the conceptualisation here, we use it in an affectionate, informal way, often to make light of ourselves. For example, if I were to go about a task in a manner that was different to the expected manner of doing that task or in a way that reflected a stereotypical autistic adherence to order and structure, my husband might sing out, 'Autie!' playfully and we'd both laugh. In the kitchen, I am very specific about what foods I will and won't handle, particularly if their preparation produces messy, slimy, smelly scraps, so I will often ask my husband to deal with these instead, which is a certain path to being called 'Autie!' In terms of my own usage of the word 'Autie,' I might refer affectionately to 'my Autie brain,' and the lightheartedness of 'Autie' here stands in firm opposition to the cold, clinical, pathologised alternatives of 'Autism spectrum disorder' or 'ASD.' 'Autie' is something that Autistic people such as myself can embrace as part of our identity. An Autistic person does things in an 'Autie' way because they – we – are Autistic. In essence, to me, 'Autie' is the recognition that my brain differs from the neuromajority – and that is perfectly okay.

Autigender 💬

Autigender describes the intersection of gender identity and autism, recognising how the unique cognitive, sensory, and social experiences of being autistic shape the way gender is experienced and expressed. For many autistic individuals, traditional concepts of gender can feel misaligned due to their sensory sensitivities and distinctive processing of social norms.

For instance, sensory sensitivities might make traditional gendered clothing uncomfortable, prompting exploration of non-gendered options for a more authentic self-expression. Autigender reframes gender identity as deeply influenced by autistic experience rather than societal expectations, challenging rigid binaries and embracing the fluid, multifaceted intersections of autism and gender as a core part of identity.

IN MY OWN WORDS: LYRIC RIVERA

Autigender is a term used to describe a person whose gender identity is deeply connected to their Autistic Experience.

This does not mean Autism is a gender. Instead, this gender label puts a focus on the influence being Autistic has on a person's experience of gender.

Disclaimer: Before I continue, it is essential to note that (like with all things), there is no unified Autistic or NeuroDivergent experience of gender.

Gender is a personal experience that can only be defined by the person experiencing it.

While I (and many other Autistic and NeuroDivergent People) feel as if their gender is influenced by their Autistic and NeuroDivergent minds, not all Autistic or NeuroDivergent People will identify with or relate to the Autigender or other NeuroGender experiences. (NeuroGender is an umbrella term describing when someone's NeuroDivergence influences their experience of gender to such a degree that they cannot separate their understanding and experience of gender).

Some might not feel that being Autistic or NeuroDivergent has an impact on their gender or their experience of gender as a social construct – and that's okay!

So, how does being NeuroDivergent, specifically Autistic, influence someone's experience of gender?

Autism influences most things in my life, including who I socialise with, my relationships, how I process information, my experience of the world around me, and my experience of gender.

Autism is tied to my hobbies, passions, interests, communication style, and habits.

Autism is interwoven into how I interpret (and fit within) social contexts, structures, and hierarchies.

That's why I say, "I am Autistic," instead of using the descriptor "person with autism" – because, for me, "with autism" minimises the impact of something so integral to nearly every aspect of my being.

Autism is NOT a separate thing that I "take with me" or something I can leave behind when I venture out into the world (even if I venture to places where being Autistic is more difficult).

Autism is not something I carry around "with me." Autism is me. If I were not Autistic, I would not be me.

Like with everything else, being Autistic has fundamentally shaped how I relate to gender. I assume this is because gender is a social construct (and social constructs are one of those things that I, like many Autistic People, don't always fit neatly within).

In my case, being Autistic means I sit outside these social constructs, examining them under a magnifying glass from afar.

I don't fit into the boxes. I make my own boxes.

I am the square peg that can't be put through the round hole (without damaging the peg) – my experience of gender is no different.

I am nonbinary (specifically genderfluid), and since I cannot separate my nonbinary experience from my Autistic, NeuroDivergent one, the labels Autigender and NeuroGender both apply (to me).

Both my NeuroDivergence and my queerness are interwoven into one another. Separating them would unravel the fabric of my existence (because they are a frame upon which my reality is built).

> My NeuroDivergent mind and my gender (which comes from the mind) are things society has pushed me to hide (because outsiders view these traits as "deviant" – diverging from a social contract I never agreed to participate in).
>
> These labels help explain my experiences, giving me back the power that was taken from me by having my experiences denied by those who forced normative expectations on me.

Autism

Autism is a neurological identity, characterising a unique way in which a person's brain and nervous system function, divergent from typical neurology. Autism is not a deficit, disorder, or anything inherently problematic or negative. Rather, it is an intrinsic part of an individual's identity, akin to ethnicity or gender, and falls within the broader spectrum of neurodiversity. Autistic individuals experience the world distinctly, with their neurological makeup shaping their sensory experience, psychology, social interactions, communication, and executive functioning.

One of the most distinguishing features of autism is hyperempathy. Contrary to common misconceptions of autistic individuals lacking empathy, autistic people can experience an intensified form of empathy, often feeling the emotions of others deeply and intensely. This heightened empathetic sensitivity is a significant and defining aspect of their social and emotional experiences. Autism also encompasses a range of sensory processing experiences, such as hypersensitivity or hyposensitivity to stimuli, influencing how autistic people interact with their surroundings. Social communication is another facet where autistic people may have their unique styles best understood and supported through neurodivergent-affirming approaches.

Understanding autism requires recognising and valuing these differences rather than perpetuating misconceptions or attempts to 'normalise' autistic individuals. Ultimately, autism is a vital aspect of human diversity, deserving respect, appreciation, and affirmation.

Autism Acceptance Month vs Autism Awareness Month

The terms 'Autism Acceptance Month' and 'Autism Awareness Month' reflect contrasting approaches to understanding and supporting the autistic community.

Autism Awareness Month is traditionally observed in April and focuses on increasing public awareness about autism. However, this approach has been increasingly criticised for perpetuating stereotypical and pathologising views of autism, often emphasising deficits rather than embracing the diversity of autistic experiences.

In contrast, Autism Acceptance Month shifts the focus to positive acknowledgement of autism as a natural variation in human neurology. It calls for societal change towards inclusivity, understanding, and valuing autistic people as they are. Moving from awareness to acceptance represents a vital step towards building a society that not only recognises autism but also respects, values and leverages the diverse needs, strengths, and experiences of autistic individuals.

IN MY OWN WORDS: WILLIAM VANDERPUYE

I used to be content with the idea of 'Autism Awareness' during my initial years of discovering and embracing my autism identity. I would order puzzle piece paraphernalia online to display around, and make social media posts daily, doubling my efforts during the month of April.

However, now I have come to believe that Awareness does not automatically constitute acceptance. Awareness means "we know you exist" Acceptance means "we value you for being you."

Numerous studies have shown that autistic people are more likely to experience suicidal ideation and Autistic people without learning disabilities are more likely to die by suicide because of lack of acceptance and a diminished sense of belonging. Symbols of autism awareness include puzzle pieces, the "light it up blue" campaign, person-first language, the medical model of disability, and the deficit model of disability. These instigate the task of curing autism, highlighting the negative aspects of autism and a focus on getting autistic people to hide their autistic traits to fit in.

On the other hand, the notion of 'Autism Acceptance' benefits autistic people as it validates us and empowers us. It gives us a sense of agency, autonomy, and acknowledgement. Autism acceptance seeks to recognise autistics not as a pathology to be cured but as a neurotype to be celebrated. Autism acceptance is at the heart of autism advocacy. Promoters of autism acceptance listen to autistic individuals and respect their chosen language, which is typically identity-first language, their preferred symbols, such as the infinity sign, and their initiatives, such as "Light It Gold."

> I also think Autism acceptance should not be merely an annual celebration but an ongoing practice to ensure the mental well-being and cohesion of autistic individuals in society.

Autism Act 2009

The Autism Act 2009 is a unique law in England, dedicated solely to autistic individuals. It aims to improve support and services for autistic adults by mandating the development of a national autism strategy to address barriers such as accessing healthcare and ensuring necessary adjustments in public services. The Act also highlighted the importance of professional training to better understand and meet the diverse needs of the autistic community.

However, critics have noted inconsistent implementation across regions, resulting in significant disparities in service provision. For example, in 2019, a report by the All-Party Parliamentary Group on Autism revealed that only 21% of councils fully comply with commitments to provide autism training for all health and care staff, and 43% lack specialist autism training for professionals conducting care assessments. These gaps illustrated that practical changes had not kept up pace with the Act's intentions, leaving many social and structural barriers unresolved.

Updates to England's autism strategy, including the 2021 strategy for autistic children, young people, and adults, have sought to address these ongoing challenges and expand the scope of support to include all age groups.

Autism parent 🚫

The term 'autism parent,' (or 'autism dad', 'autism mom/mum'), often used by parents of autistic individuals, is problematic because it centres on the experiences of parents rather than the autistic people themselves, potentially overshadowing their voices, needs, and experiences. This framing can reinforce narratives that portray autism primarily as a burden or challenge rather than as a legitimate and valuable neurological identity. Additionally, the term oversimplifies a diverse group of parents with varying experiences, failing to capture the complexity of their roles. Instead, phrasing like 'parent of an autistic person' acknowledges the autonomy and personhood of autistic individuals while promoting dignity, inclusion, and a more respectful perspective.

Autism spectrum condition 💬 🚫

The term 'autism spectrum condition' (ASC) represents a move away from the highly pathologising term 'autism spectrum disorder' (ASD). While it offers some improvement, it still subtly frames autism as a medical condition rather than a natural and valid aspect of human diversity.

A more affirming approach is to use terms like autism or autistic, recognising these as part of a person's neurological identity rather than a 'condition' or 'disorder.' This perspective views autism as a natural variation in human neurology, akin to other aspects of identity such as gender or ethnicity. It highlights the importance of embracing and valuing the unique experiences, strengths, and challenges that come with being autistic.

Autism spectrum disorder

The term 'autism spectrum disorder' (ASD) is deeply problematic due to its pathologising connotations. It frames autism as a disorder requiring treatment, which contradicts the neurodiversity perspective that recognises autism as a natural neurological variation and identity. The use of 'ASD' in clinical and diagnostic settings often fuels stigma and misunderstanding, contributing to negative stereotypes about autistic individuals.

For example, labelling autism as a 'disorder' can lead to assumptions that autistic people inherently struggle or lack abilities, overshadowing their strengths and unique perspectives. This misconception can lower expectations and limit opportunities in education, employment, and social interactions.

Advocates of neurodiversity promote using terms like autism or autistic, which honour the identity of autistic individuals, and emphasise societal acceptance, inclusion, and respect.

Autism stigma

Autism stigma refers to the harmful stereotypes, discrimination, and social labelling directed towards autistic people and, at times, their families. This can manifest as 'public stigma' or 'social stigma,' where society views autism negatively, or as 'courtesy stigma' (also known as 'associative' or 'family stigma'), which affects the relatives or close associates of autistic individuals. Stigma may also stem from professionals in health, education, and social services ('professional' or 'structural stigma'). When autistic people internalise these negative views, it is termed 'self-stigma' or 'internalised stigma.' A related concept, 'affiliate stigma,' occurs when family carers internalise negative beliefs about autism. All forms of autism stigma can have serious consequences, including worsening mental health, contributing to depression, anxiety, distress, and even suicidal ideation. The expression of autism stigma varies across different social and cultural contexts.

Autistic community ⚖️

The autistic community is a collective of autistic individuals united by shared neurological identity, mutual understanding, and a sense of belonging. Far from being monolithic, the autistic community reflects the diversity of autism itself, positively and safely embracing a wide range of perspectives and experiences. This community transcends geographical boundaries and focuses on connecting through common experiences, knowledge exchange, mutual support, and collective advocacy for autism acceptance and rights.

IN MY OWN WORDS: ADITI GANGRADE

I've always felt like an imposter.

During most of my teenage years, I kept asking myself, "Why am I different from my peers?" I couldn't quite pinpoint what it was, but I just knew I didn't fit in. It felt like I had to put in extra effort to be included, whether it was with classmates or kids in the neighborhood.

Socializing seemed so natural for everyone else – it just happened, without effort. But even though I loved talking to people and making new friends, I kept hearing words like "oversensitive," "too serious," or even "weird" when it came to me.

I learned, silently and subconsciously, that my natural reactions and behaviors weren't accepted. The reason I was left out of plans or groups was because I didn't fit the mold.

Growing up in a collectivist culture like India's, doing things alone wasn't seen as "normal."

You were supposed to fit in, belong to a group, be part of a community. And while India's culture is incredibly diverse, I noticed something early on: I wasn't the only one struggling to fit in. Other kids had similar challenges, not because they were neurodivergent, but because of their looks – skin color, facial features – or their social status, religion, caste, popularity, or disability.

With those kids, I didn't feel so strange. I could be myself around them.

Even though I had to learn how to mask to survive as a girl in India, there were one or two people who made me feel at home. Our friendships were different. We didn't hang out all the time, didn't have a group, and we'd talk maybe once or twice a month. But we were there for each other, and that was enough.

That's when I first found a sense of community.

Knowing that there's someone out there who gets you, who makes you feel like you're not alone – that feeling means everything.

So, after my partner and I both discovered our neurodivergence, we felt a strong need for community. And that's how Much Much Spectrum came to life, part of our media company, Much Much Media.

While we started making films and content on firsthand lived experiences through our company, extended family, relatives, and friends started distancing themselves from us. Some didn't know what being neurodivergent meant and so stopped hanging out that often.

I have often felt like an imposter while talking about myself. Not being able to articulate myself brought immense shame.

When people saw my films and work, they would have a certain image of me in their head (which was often really good), but I felt like as soon as they met me that image just shattered. They took me lightly and the respect they had for me earlier would seem to decline. And that just messed a lot with my mental health and self-image.

But we found new people through the Much Much Spectrum community – who opened their arms to embrace us.

Any human rights movement thrives when people come together to uplift one another and take action. Over the last two years, I've seen how autistic communities have flourished, especially online.

In neurodivergent spaces, there's warmth, acceptance, and support.

We can be ourselves, stand up for ourselves, shed the shame, and take pride in being different. I feel understood without having to explain or hide parts of myself.

On my worst days – when I've struggled with anger or grief about my disability – I've found love and care from the Much Much Spectrum community.

It's not just my incredibly supportive partner; it's the people who show up, hold space for me, and connect with the stories I share.

This community has given me confidence I didn't know I had. Together, we've built a 60k-strong global audience, made resources more accessible, and are redefining what "normal" means, one story at a time.

Autistic flow

Autistic flow refers to a distinct state of intense focus and immersion that autistic individuals often experience when engaging with activities that deeply resonate with their interests or passions. This phenomenon is akin to the broader psychological concept of 'flow,' yet it manifests uniquely within the autistic context. Autistic individuals might find themselves completely absorbed in a task, losing track of time and external distractions, which can lead to profound satisfaction and a sense of accomplishment. This state is not only indicative of the deep, intrinsic motivation driving the individual but also highlights the exceptional capacity for concentration and dedication.

IN MY OWN WORDS: AGUSTINA CARDOSO

Autistic flow, for me, isn't just about focus; it's a haven where my busy mind finally finds peace and quiet. The usual whirlwind of thoughts slows down, and I enter a realm of mental silence. It's in this space that I experience a deep sense of contentment and joy, one that I can't access otherwise. Tasks that might feel difficult or draining in other contexts become almost effortless. It's as if my mind and my chosen activity become totally in sync, and everything simply flows organically. It's like my brain takes a deep breath.

But perhaps the most remarkable aspect of autistic flow is its ability to provide a sense of refuge from the chaos of the outside world. In a society that often feels overwhelming and unpredictable, this state offers safety, a place without judgment or misunderstanding. And while autistic flow is not always easy to achieve, as it requires the right conditions – quiet surroundings, familiar routines, and the absence of external pressures – when everything aligns, the rewards are immeasurable.

By allowing ourselves the space to reach these flow states, we provide ourselves with an extraordinary tool to self-regulate and recover when the world becomes too much.

Autistic inertia

Autistic inertia refers to a phenomenon often observed in autistic people, characterised by a pronounced preference to maintain their current state of activity or inactivity. This concept suggests that an autistic person may remain in their existing state – either at rest or in motion – until there is a prompt for change.

For example, an autistic person might find it difficult to start a task like washing the dishes, even if they recognise it needs to be done. Once they begin, however, they might find it equally challenging to stop, becoming deeply focused and continuing to clean far beyond the initial task. This inertia is not a choice or a lack of will but a significant aspect of autistic neurology. Recognising and understanding autistic inertia emphasises the importance of patience and tailored support, such as breaking tasks into smaller steps or using gentle prompts, to facilitate smoother transitions for autistic people.

IN MY OWN WORDS: AGUSTINA CARDOSO

Autistic inertia feels like being glued to my current state of activity or inactivity. It's as if my mind and body are separate entities, and I can't move forward, and I can't move backward, no matter how hard I want to do it.

The impact of autistic inertia on mental health, especially for late-diagnosed neurodivergent people like myself, cannot be overstated. Navigating a world designed for neurotypical brains is already challenging in its own right, but when you add the weight of autistic inertia to the mix, it can feel like constantly swimming against the current.

I spent years struggling to understand why I couldn't "simply do it" like everyone else seemed to be able to do. There were countless moments when I gave myself a hard time for not being able to force my brain to cooperate with what I had to do, even with what I wanted to do. It's easy to internalise these struggles as personal failures, as if something is fundamentally wrong with the way your brain works.

Understanding and recognising autistic inertia is crucial because it highlights the need for patience and tailored support to navigate task management and transitions effectively. And it's key to recognise it not as a personal failing, but as a natural aspect of our neurotype.

Autistic language hypothesis

The autistic language hypothesis posits that autistic communication styles are distinct, valid, and natural variations in human communication, not deficiencies or disorders. It challenges the view that differences in language use are inherently problematic, advocating for greater understanding and acceptance of these unique patterns.

Autistic individuals may prefer direct, unambiguous language, written over verbal communication, or alternative approaches to non-speaking cues like eye contact. For example, echolalia – the repetition of phrases – is often a meaningful way to express thoughts or process information rather than mere mimicry.

This hypothesis emphasises that communication challenges stem not from autistic communication itself, but from the mismatch between autistic and neurotypical styles.

IN MY OWN WORDS: JORIS FOUET

I don't understand lyrics in songs. I'll hear it, I'll focus on it, I'll enjoy it, but if it were Swedish I would have the same experience. And indeed, I listen to Japanese pop exactly the same way I do English singer-songwriters: following melodies.

That's because in music, the smallest unit of meaning is not a tone; it's a melody. It's how it ends contrasting with how it started. Half a melody begs to be finished. And you won't know if you like it until it does. One key tenet of the autistic language hypothesis is that neurotypical people process semantic meaning at the sentence level, and autistic people break it down further: words, or even syllables, carry their own, full, self-contained meaning and need to be processed as such.

And indeed, I don't ascribe meaning to a sentence that isn't the sum of its parts. i.e. I don't do metaphors.

Now, with all that said, if I listen to lyrics I like, and I break it down consciously into bits, and recreate a sentence without the melody, only then do I hear separate words and semantic meaning emerges. I literally have to repeat the lyrics back to myself to understand them.

But I do understand them!

When talking with other people, we are clearly talking about the same thing. It just takes some specific processing for me to get there.

Autistic-led ⚖️

The term 'autistic-led' refers to an approach where communities, research, support, representation, and training related to autistic people are directed and led by autistic individuals themselves. This approach recognises that autistic people are uniquely qualified to understand and advocate for their own needs and experiences, making it not just a valid choice but the most ethical and effective way to address issues impacting their lives. By prioritising autistic leadership, this model not only enhances representation but also enriches the wider community's understanding and acceptance of autistic culture.

Autistic-led identity support ⚖️ 🛡️

Autistic-led identity support refers to peer-led support by autistic individuals, focused on empowering a positive autistic identity. This approach supports autistic people to embrace their neurodivergent identity authentically, in contrast to traditional interventions that often prioritise conformity to neurotypical norms.

The effectiveness of this support stems from the safety and insight unique to shared autistic experiences. Being in a space where the support is led by someone who is also autistic creates a sense of safety, free from judgement or misunderstanding. This mutual understanding enables a deep sense of belonging and validation.

This form of support is particularly valuable for neurodivergent individuals who are newly discovering their identity and beginning their journey of self-understanding and acceptance, as well as for those working to resist and reject internalised ableism.

Autistic-led mental health therapy ⚖️ 🛡️

Autistic-led mental health therapy involves mental health professionals, who are themselves autistic, providing therapy to autistic clients. This approach greatly enhances the therapeutic process, with the shared experience of being autistic enables a deeper connection and trust between therapist and client, crucial for effective therapy. Autistic therapists are ideally placed to offer strategies that resonate with autistic ways of thinking and feeling rather than applying standard neurotypical models. This approach not only empowers clients but also challenges traditional mental health paradigms, highlighting the value of diversity in mental health professionals. However, the availability of autistic-led therapy and its recognition in mainstream mental health services are issues that require development.

IN MY OWN WORDS: ANDREW KINGSLOW

First, I think it's best to speak about my experiences before discovering Autistic-Led Therapy, as they highlight the issues I faced and how traditional therapy often worsened my mental state. I have undergone various periods of therapy, mostly comprising cognitive behavioural therapy (CBT). I found CBT triggering, traumatic, and frustrating due to its focus on feelings and thoughts. Although I hadn't been diagnosed at the time, I struggled intensely with this form of therapy. In retrospect, I realise that my difficulty was due to Alexithymia, which led me to speak from an analytical mindset and essentially mask my way through sessions. Often, I left sessions triggered and occasionally in a state of meltdown. As an autistic individual, reliving past trauma can feel as intense as when it first happened. Even as I write this, those same feelings are stirring within me, so I will move on swiftly.

Autistic-Led Therapy came to me in the form of identity therapy. It was the first time I spoke to someone with a common ground, and I didn't feel pathologised. The peculiarities I was told made me different, awkward, or eccentric were part of a neurotype and, by extension, part of a community that understood each other. I soon discovered that my therapist and I shared real-world experiences, which was a watershed moment. I no longer felt alone in my experience. Having my mental dissonance contextualised and explained in a clinical way appealed to my logical brain and provided closure on a myriad of unanswered questions.

It is absolutely imperative that neurodivergent individuals have access to therapists and counsellors who can interact and empathise directly. There is a hidden sixth, seventh, or even eighth sense that comes into play in the relationship, one that builds trust through true empathy and actual understanding. It's much easier to open the doors of the mind when there's someone like-minded holding your hand.

Autistic pride ⚖️ 🛡️

Autistic pride is an ideology that celebrates the unique attributes and perspectives of autistic individuals, advocating for the recognition of autism as a natural variation in human neurocognition. It challenges the traditional deficit-focused view of autism, promoting self-acceptance and positive identity among autistic people.

Autistic pride events bring this ideology into action, transforming it into a tangible and communal experience. These gatherings provide a space where autistic individuals can come together to celebrate their identity, share their stories, and showcase their talents. By operationalising the principles of autistic pride, these events not only affirm self-acceptance within the autistic community but also increase public understanding and acceptance of autism.

Autonomous sensory meridian response

Autonomous sensory meridian response (ASMR) refers to a unique sensory phenomenon experienced by some people, characterised by a tingling sensation that usually starts on the scalp and moves down the spine. Triggered by auditory or visual stimuli such as whispering, tapping, or soft repetitive sounds, ASMR can create a calming, pleasurable, or even deeply relaxing experience for individuals. It has gained attention in recent years through online content that aims to elicit these responses, often being described as soothing or stress-relieving. ASMR content can be particularly beneficial for some autistic people, offering calming sensory input or aiding in sensory regulation. However, sensory perception is highly individualised, and what is soothing for one person may be overstimulating or uncomfortable for another.

Autonomy

Autonomy emphasises the right of autistic and other neurodivergent individuals to self-governance and to make decisions independently. This concept is fundamental in recognising and respecting the individuality and agency of neurodivergent people. Autonomy challenges the often paternalistic approaches in traditional support systems where decisions are made for rather than with, neurodivergent individuals. In enabling autonomy, the focus shifts from an imposed standard of 'normalcy' to embracing the diverse ways in which autistic and other neurodivergent people interact with and perceive the world. This empowerment is vital for the well-being and self-determination of such people, ensuring their voices are central in all matters concerning their lives.

Autopia

'Autopia' is a conceptual term that represents an idealised vision or society where autistic individuals can live and thrive as equals, fully respected for their neurodivergent nature. In autopia, societal norms, environments, and systems are designed to be inherently inclusive. Therefore, autopia represents a goal where autistic people can experience full participation, equality, and acceptance, with their contributions recognised and valued as part of the rich tapestry of human diversity.

Avoidant/restrictive food intake disorder

Avoidant/restrictive food intake disorder (ARFID) is an eating challenge characterised by profound avoidance or restriction of food intake, unrelated to body image concerns. It often stems from sensory sensitivities, adverse eating experiences, or anxiety surrounding food. This is particularly common among autistic individuals, where strong aversions to textures, colours, tastes, or environments can cause extreme selectivity or distress around eating.

ARFID can result in significant nutritional deficits and social difficulties, as affected individuals may struggle to eat in typical social settings. Addressing ARFID in neurodivergent people requires a neurodivergent-affirming approach, such as trauma-informed care that validates individual needs rather than pathologising behaviours.

Support strategies include co-regulation and sensory safety, where a trusted partner (like a caregiver) responds empathetically to the individual's needs. For example, if the texture of food is overwhelming, the caregiver might sit with them during meals, modelling calm, positive interactions with food, such as exploring or smelling new items without pressure to eat. This builds trust, reduces anxiety, and allows the individual to engage with food at their own pace in a supportive environment.

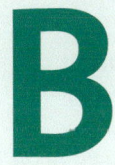

Behaviours that challenge 💬

'Behaviours that challenge' reframes the pathologising view of 'challenging behaviours' in autistic people. It recognises that what may be perceived as challenging is often a reflection of the discordance between the individual's needs and their environment. Therefore, unlike the term 'challenging behaviours,' the term underscores that these behaviours are not inherently problematic but are responses to external stimuli and/or internal states. It also challenges the notion of pathologising autistic behaviours, advocating for environments and approaches that are respectful and neurodivergent-affirming. This perspective encourages a deeper exploration of the root causes of these behaviours, promoting acceptance and accommodation over traditional views that seek to modify or suppress them.

Binaural sound therapy 🌿 💧

Binaural sound therapy involves listening to sounds of differing frequencies in each ear, creating a perceived auditory beat, or binaural beat, within the brain. This phenomenon is thought to influence brainwave activity, promoting mental states like relaxation, improved focus, or altered consciousness. Specific frequency combinations are claimed to reduce anxiety, enhance sleep, and boost mental clarity. However, evidence for its efficacy is mixed, with some suggesting its effects may stem from placebo rather than the therapy itself. While it is non-invasive and easily accessible through headphones or speakers, its benefits should not be overstated without stronger empirical support.

Bipolar 💬 🌿

Bipolar, or bipolar disorder, encompassing Bipolar I and II, is characterised by significant mood variations. Bipolar I involves pronounced manic episodes, often leading to intense highs, contrasted with depressive periods. Bipolar II features less severe hypomanic episodes coupled with significant depressive episodes. While typically classified as a mood disorder, bipolar also represents a deviation from neurotypical cognition and is integral to an individual's identity and experience, aligning with broader neurodiversity principles.

DOI: 10.4324/9781003477297-2

Body doubling 👥 🧍 🏢

Body doubling is a supportive strategy for enhancing focus and productivity. It involves the presence of another person working alongside the individual, not necessarily on the same task, but providing a subtle social framework that can help in mitigating distractions and maintaining focus. The presence of another can be a calming, grounding influence, particularly for those who might struggle with executive functioning challenges such as initiating tasks, sustaining attention, or managing time effectively. This concept challenges traditional notions of independence, emphasising the neurodivergent-affirming principle that interdependence can be a strength. It also highlights the importance of adopting innovative, personalised support strategies for neurodivergent individuals in personal and professional contexts.

IN MY OWN WORDS: AGUSTINA CARDOSO

Body doubling is like having a silent accountability partner. It helps me create a dedicated workspace and time, making it easier to resist distractions. There's something about having someone present, even if we're not interacting much – or even at all– that motivates me to stay on task to honour my commitment to the work I'm doing because I'm not doing it just for myself, it involves someone else now.

The tendency to become easily distracted or overwhelmed can make starting and finishing tasks very challenging. Body doubling offers me a structured context where the mere presence of another person can reduce the impulse to stray from the task at hand, especially when things have become overwhelming or I'm suddenly stuck with what to do next. It can also offer a sense of routine for me as it allows a stable environment that helps mitigate the anxiety and sensory overload (that sometimes comes from lack of sensory stimuli) often associated with working alone.

This person offers moral support and encouragement without even being aware of it, making the often-daunting tasks of working or studying alone feel more manageable and less isolating as a result. Emotionally, it can also provide comfort without the need for direct social interaction, which can sometimes be draining.

Body doubling has been incredibly beneficial for me, and I believe it has played a crucial role in my academic performance. I don't think I would've been able to go through my college assignment load without resorting to body doubling, either with classmates or even my mum or partner. The beauty of body doubling is that it doesn't require a shared task. It's not about the specific work you're doing; it's about both people being on the same wavelength and work mindset so that you can see the task through to completion.

Essentially, body doubling provides a sense of camaraderie and accountability that transforms the isolating and often overwhelming experience of working or studying alone into something more manageable and even enjoyable.

Brain-computer interfaces

Brain-computer interfaces (BCIs) are tools that translate brain signals into commands, enabling non-speaking individuals to communicate and interact with their environment without traditional speech or manual input.

While BCIs hold promise, their development and use must prioritise the dignity, consent, and individuality of the user. They should complement, not replace, less invasive communication tools like picture boards, and must never serve as an excuse to neglect creating supportive environments for non-speakers.

As this technology is still in its infancy, research must be guided by the non-speaking neurodivergent community to ensure ethical and appropriate use. BCIs should only be implemented with the informed consent of the individual, free from pressure or coercion, respecting their right to choose how they communicate and engage with the world.

Bruxism

Bruxism, commonly known as teeth grinding, arises from unique sensory processing, stress coping mechanisms, or as a non-speaking communication method with non-speaking people potentially using teeth grinding to express discomfort or frustration. Sensory sensitivities might lead to the grinding of teeth as a way of managing such sensations or seeking comfort making teeth grinding a form of self-regulation akin to stimming. Understanding the underlying reasons for bruxism, such as the potential environmental or sensory-based stressors, is key for support.

Bullying

Bullying involves repeated and intentional harm directed at an individual or group, often manifesting through physical, verbal, psychological, social, or sexual aggression. It is prevalent in various settings, such as schools, workplaces, and online platforms, and disproportionately affects neurodivergent individuals. Its impact is profound and far-reaching, harming mental health, self-esteem, and overall well-being, with long-term consequences including an elevated risk of suicidal ideation.

The motivations of bullies stem from a myriad of factors, including a lack of understanding and acceptance of neurodivergence leading to discrimination against those who diverge from societal norms, a desire for control, or mirroring behaviour seen in their own environments. In some cases, bullying is a misguided effort to enhance their own sense of worth or competence, particularly if they are struggling with insecurities or personal challenges. Addressing bullying requires comprehensive strategies that target its root causes and create empathy and respect for neurodivergence at both individual and systemic levels.

Burnout 🗨️ 🌿 🚫

Neurodivergent people often face a significant risk of burnout, a state of intense mental, physical, or emotional exhaustion resulting from prolonged use of cognitive and psychological coping strategies, whether conscious, sub-conscious or unconscious, in response to chronically demanding situations. Autistic burnout is characterised by overwhelming fatigue, reduced performance, and a diminished sense of personal accomplishment. It is worsened by the effort to conform to a neurotypical world and mask natural autistic traits. The implications of burnout can be severe including less ability to manage and cope with daily life and deteriorated mental health.

Mitigating against burnout requires a substantial social, cultural, and systemic shift that fully allows, accepts, and supports neurodivergent people to be themselves, eliminating the need for masking. Compassionate understanding and analysis of contributing factors are essential to support recovery and prevent future occurrences.

IN MY OWN WORDS: BEN BREAUX

In my experience, non-speaking burnout is different from speakers. My impulses become harder to control and I seem to be overflowing with energy. However, this couldn't be further from the truth. On the outside, I will seem happy, but I am masking. Oftentimes my masking is unintentional. I appear energized – I will jump around with my smile at full power. This is an attempt at regulating. So many people see this and think this means they can ask me to do more but that just makes everything worse. It feels like endless stress and the inability to recoup. It also becomes hard to control my body in these moments, which just increases the stress. It feels like all the pressure of the world is suffocating me.

Occasionally, I feel pressure to participate in the neurotypical world and mask my burnout; I especially do this for certain people – people who don't know what autism really is. It's hard to interact with people that don't understand – it only serves to push me further into burnout territory. Being around people that accept me alleviates the stress and potential for burnout.

The neurotypical world is so loud and bright. It takes so much energy to function. Usually I can interact in this world with minimal issues with some exceptions, such as food. However, some situations are just too much. This can include shopping malls or theme parks when they're crowded. Sensations like heat and physical touch or proximity can almost be painful at times. Neurotypicals can find this hard to understand and it can overwhelm me.

I need frequent breaks from work to avoid burnout. It helps when people can read my body language. So, intuitive people are usually my go-to. Fidgets are also helpful for every day regulation so I don't burn out as easily. It can be hard to get back from a state of burnout; usually it takes me a few days to recover. I typically need relaxation and time away from work.

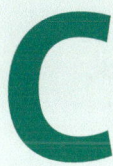

Camouflaging

Camouflaging is psychological, adaptive strategy where autistic people alter their natural behaviours, expressions, or reactions to conform to societal norms or expectations. This conscious or subconscious effort to mask autistic traits, driven by the desire for acceptance, safety, or smoother social interactions, may facilitate short-term integration but comes with significant psychological costs. Sustained camouflaging increases stress, exhaustion, and the risk of mental health issues such as anxiety and depression.

The societal pressures that make camouflaging necessary need to be challenged, with a focus on creating environments where autistic people can feel able to express their neurodivergence authentically and without fear of repercussions.

IN MY OWN WORDS: LYRIC RIVERA

Neurodivergent camouflaging refers to the strategies and coping mechanisms employed by NeuroDivergent People to tone down, conceal, or mask our NeuroDivergent traits when engaging in spaces or with people that make us feel guarded due to a lack of (or perceived lack of) emotional and/or physical safety.

This camouflaging can manifest in various ways, such as continued self-monitoring and analysis to emulate and mimic neuro-normative behaviors (even if they feel unnatural and foreign to us), suppressing natural responses and adopting socially acceptable mannerisms.

We may also work on toning down our NeuroDivergent traits to avoid standing out or being perceived as different (because doing so can have serious, sometimes dangerous, consequences).

For instance, an Autistic Person might force themselves to make eye contact, hide their special interests, or imitate social interactions they've observed

DOI: 10.4324/9781003477297-3

(and possibly studied). Or you may have a person in a group who, despite being passionate or well-informed about a topic, holds themselves back, refraining from sharing their knowledge or enthusiasm (to avoid being judged).

Camouflaging, for many NeuroDivergent People, is not a choice but a necessity (driven by the fear of judgment, rejection, or even harm). It can be exhausting and anxiety-provoking, as NeuroDivergent People may feel as if we need to constantly monitor and adjust ourselves to avoid harsh (unsolicited) reviews and criticisms from the people around us. This exhaustion can be even more extreme for multiply-NeuroDivergent individuals and NeuroDivergent People who are multiply marginalized, as having numerous identities that society dismisses can create additional pressure to mask or hide parts of oneself.

The more parts you try to hide, the more burden you may feel from the weight of blending in (especially for those of us who feel forced to hide parts of ourselves we cannot conceal).

Camouflaging can be done consciously, meaning we may be aware of our effort to conform, or it may become so ingrained in us that we camouflage ourselves subconsciously (without realizing we are doing it) – especially when we feel unsafe. Blending in is a survival skill we develop to protect ourselves. And for many of us, camouflaging is a trauma response.

Though physically and mentally exhausting, camouflaging had become second nature to me.

I learned to hide my weaknesses (by never asking for help).

I compensated for my spoken communication difficulties by spending extra time preparing and rehearsing conversations, writing up complex, scripted responses and literal scripts (that I would rehearse and then read for phone calls and other meetings).

Not only did I hide my weaknesses and difficulties, but I also hid my strengths, hobbies, interests, and passions (if they drew too much attention).

I found ways to compensate for (or mask) my struggles and differences (and sometimes even my joy and happiness), but not all NeuroDivergent People can hide how they are different.

For those who do camouflage ourselves, this ability to hide may fluctuate throughout a person's lifetime (or even day-to-day).

Because many of us cannot camouflage at all or may not be able to blend in at all times, we need the world to be (emotionally and physically) safer for those of us who are more vulnerable (because of how we stand out).

By creating safe spaces where NeuroDivergent People can openly express ourselves (without fear of judgment or rejection), we can break down the barriers that force us to hide ourselves (and our needs) from those around us.

Care Act 2014 ⚖

A significant piece of legislation in England, the Care Act 2014 is designed to enhance care and support by focusing on individual well-being, personalised care, and accessibility. It promotes a strengths-based approach, emphasising individual capabilities and tailoring support plans to personal needs and outcomes. Local authorities are required to assess and meet the eligible needs of adults, including autistic individuals, moving away from one-size-fits-all solutions. The Act also seeks to reduce social isolation; strengthen community ties; and uphold dignity, rights, and inclusion while recognising and supporting the essential role of carers.

However, the Act's implementation has faced challenges. Funding shortfalls have led to inconsistent delivery across local authorities, leaving many autistic individuals and those with complex needs without timely or reliable support. Budget cuts to social care have further weakened its effectiveness, and carers often feel under-supported despite their rights.

While updates have aimed to improve integration with health services and safeguarding, funding gaps and poor coordination remain significant obstacles. Many argue that broader reforms are needed for the Act to achieve its full potential.

IN MY OWN WORDS: WILLIAM VANDERPUYE

The room was poorly lit except for a slight slit in the curtains that ushered in a comforting ray of sunshine. Although the house was clean, hoards of utensils, books, video tapes, and furniture gave the otherwise spacious room a feeling of chaos and claustrophobia. An elderly lady sat in a reclining chair in the centre of the room. She had turned off the television for our meeting.

This was to be the first Care Act Assessment I was conducting independently as a student, having shadowed countless similar assessments. As a social worker who has now worked in adult mental health and learning disabilities, the Care Act 2014 is a major piece of legislation that governs my daily tasks.

Doreen (not her real name) talked extensively about her day from when she woke to when she retired to bed, as I listened intently and followed up with prompts. She spoke about how difficult it was to get up from bed in the morning due to ongoing bodily pains which forced her to hold unto furniture to mobilise (known as furniture-walking). She spoke about her risk of falling in the bathroom, her difficulties with preparing food at mealtimes, and how difficult it is for her to do the laundry. We left no stone unturned as we explored her ability to independently use the toilet, self-medicate, undertake repairs in the home, and dress appropriately. I encouraged her to tell me about what she could do for herself, as per the strength-based practice.

Then we delved into her aspirations, her social life. Doreen revealed that in the past she ran a pub with her late husband and it was a very lucrative business at the time. She had lots of friends and acquaintances to speak to every day, and all of a sudden, she feels like her entire life has been taken away from her: all she has is the TV for company and the sight of the four walls in the living room of her ground floor one bedroom apartment. She stated that she would love to be able to go out and meet people, play bridge or bingo.

As I exited Doreen's company to compile the Care Act assessment, I realised the importance of this piece of legislation and how it helped to highlight not the problem but the person behind the problem. The Individual behind the intervention. The Care Act assessment highlighted aspects of Doreen's identity that were not immediately obvious. When the case was first allocated to me, Doreen was just an elderly person with a case number and a cocktail of conditions: diabetes, depression, and potentially dementia. When I first met her, she was an elderly lady with poor mobility in a crowded environment. By the time I left her home, Doreen was no longer a total stranger with a list of conditions. She was a mother and a bubbly, chatty former pub land lady who valued her autonomy and independence. She had fond memories of her past and her husband. She would brighten up as she shared stories of the war, displayed sepia pictures of defunct loved ones. I had enough information to put together a person-centered assessment and a personalised support plan that takes into account her strengths, her likes, and her wishes.

The Care Act places the responsibility upon the local authority to assess individuals with care and support needs and to fund appropriate interventions to meet their eligible needs. Doreen was eventually granted a package of care that included an Occupational Therapy assessment and intervention to address her furniture walking, support to attend a day centre to prevent social isolation, and assistive technology to alert professionals if she becomes unwell or falls.

Celebration ⚖️

Celebration, in the context of neurodiversity, encompasses the recognition and appreciation of the inherent value and contributions of neurodivergent individuals to society. It is a positive framing that encourages a shift from viewing neurodivergence as a deviation needing correction to understanding it as a natural and valuable variation within the human condition. Celebrating neurodivergence involves not only individual achievements but also the broader acceptance and integration of neurodivergent ways of being into all areas of societal life, including education, employment, and social policies. It advocates for environments that not only accommodate but also embrace different neurological makeups, creating a culture where all individuals can thrive without the need to camouflage their true selves.

Challenging behaviour 🚫

Challenging behaviour traditionally refers to actions by neurodivergent individuals seen as problematic in social, educational, or healthcare settings. However, this perspective is deeply flawed, as it implies these behaviours are inherently problematic rather than recognising them as communication-based responses to unmet needs, distress, stigma, or environmental mismatches. Viewing these behaviours as inherently problematic reflects a reductive approach that dismisses the critical examination of environmental factors prompting them. While investigating these factors requires effort, it is essential. Automatically attributing the issue to the individual rather than the environment stems from stigma and misunderstanding, perpetuating the harmful assumption that neurodivergent or autistic behaviours are the problem rather than the circumstances surrounding them.

Children and Families Act 2014 ⚖️

The Children and Families Act 2014 is a law in England designed to improve support for children and young people with special educational needs and disabilities (SEND), along with their families. It introduced Education, Health, and Care plans (EHCPs) to provide integrated, tailored assistance through collaboration among health, education, and social care services.

For autistic children, the Act promotes inclusion and addresses individual needs in schools. A student experiencing sensory overload might receive an EHCP detailing accommodations such as sensory breaks, access to quiet spaces, or support from a teaching assistant. Schools, health practitioners, and local authorities would then be responsible for implementing and reviewing these measures to enhance the child's learning experience and well-being.

Critics have noted regional inconsistencies in the Act's application, often due to resource shortages and inadequate training, leading to delays and uneven support. Despite amendments aimed at strengthening EHCPs and improving service coordination, significant gaps in provision and disparities in outcomes for children with SEND remain ongoing challenges.

Chronagnosia

Often called 'time blindness,' chronagnosia is a neurological phenomenon common in the neurodivergent community, involving difficulties perceiving, estimating, or managing time. People with chronagnosia may find it difficult to meet deadlines, be punctual, or organise tasks – not out of negligence or forgetfulness, but due to their unique neurocognitive wiring that deviates from the typical sense of time.

Chronagnosia challenges societal expectations of a uniform experience of time, emphasising the need for accommodations that respect diverse time-processing styles. Understanding and supporting chronagnosia can enable neurodivergent individuals to thrive beyond traditional temporal frameworks.

IN MY OWN WORDS: AGUSTINA CARDOSO

Living with chronagnosia, or time blindness, is like navigating a world where the usual markers of time are blurred and unreliable. Imagine trying to follow a schedule in a place where the time on your watch changes unpredictably and doesn't match the actual hour. At one moment, it feels like it's 3 p.m – you're full of energy and ready for afternoon tasks – only to find out that it's actually 7 p.m. and the day is almost over. Later, 7 p.m. feels like 10 p.m., and you're confused why you're not in bed yet.

In essence, it's like having your internal clock set to a different time zone that shifts constantly. You can't rely on your sense of time to guide your day, so you must make a conscious effort to track time, much like constantly checking a map in an unfamiliar city because the landmarks don't look familiar. Your internal sense of how long things take or what time it should be at a given moment is skewed, requiring you to constantly adjust and reorient yourself to match the reality around you.

In practical terms, this means I'm often late or sometimes chronically early because my sense of when I should do certain things is unreliable. I'm absolutely terrible at estimating how long tasks will take me, leading me to either overestimate and postpone them or underestimate and find myself rushing in the last minute, stressed and anxious about it.

Time management is a significant challenge because my internal clock doesn't match the actual time, but it can easily become an emotion dysregulation trigger for me. This constant need to check and recheck the time in order to meet demands can be daunting when you become painstakingly aware of how much time you spend on even the tiniest tasks. I've found myself obsessing over how fast time is passing by, how much time I'm "wasting" on simple human-related tasks like making food, showering, even sleeping. What starts as "I'm sometimes super late" can slowly turn into an existential crisis as a result of feeling trapped in a constant battle against time, leading to a sense of disconnection from yourself and the world around you.

Classroom adjustments

Classroom adjustments involve modifications and tools designed to create inclusive environments that support the diverse needs of all students, including neurodivergent learners. These adjustments remove barriers to learning and participation, ensuring every student can access the curriculum and engage fully. Examples include tailored teaching strategies, assistive technology, flexible seating arrangements, and sensory friendly changes such as adjustments to lighting or noise levels.

Sensory items are a vital part of these adjustments, aiding focus and reducing anxiety. Tools like fidget devices, such as stress balls and spinners, provide tactile outlets for energy, while weighted lap pads and blankets offer comforting pressure to enhance security. Noise-cancelling headphones or earplugs help students sensitive to auditory stimuli by creating a quieter environment, and textured tactile mats or tapes discreetly provide sensory input under desks.

Visual timers and clocks assist with time management and reduce anxiety during transitions, while chewelry (chewable jewellery) supports oral sensory needs, promoting self-regulation. Aromatherapy diffusers introduce calming scents for a soothing atmosphere, and seat cushions or discs allow subtle movement to improve concentration. Additionally, liquid timers and other calming visual stimuli help students regulate emotions and maintain focus.

These adjustments and tools are essential components of an equitable education system. By creating environments that value diverse learning and sensory profiles, they ensure that all students, especially neurodivergent ones, have the opportunity to thrive and succeed.

Code-switching

Code-switching involves adapting one's communication style to align with dominant cultural or social norms, often to ensure safety, respect, or access to opportunities. This reflects systemic pressures to suppress aspects of identity in spaces controlled by those in power. While commonly associated with ethnic and cultural minorities adjusting to white-majority norms, it extends to other dynamics, such as non-male individuals navigating male-dominated cultures.

For autistic people, particularly those with intersecting identities, this means navigating multiple pressures to conform: altering their communication to meet both neurotypical and other dominant norms. This intersectional code-switching compounds the challenges of being expected to mask autistic traits to mimic neurotypical social behaviours. While both code-switching and autistic masking involve adapting oneself to fit expected norms, the motivations and experiences differ; masking centres on reducing the visibility of autistic traits, whereas code-switching addresses broader cultural assimilation and survival.

Cognitive behavioural therapy

Cognitive behavioural therapy (CBT), developed within a neurotypical framework, is unsuitable for many autistic and neurodivergent individuals. Its foundations and research are predominantly neurotypical-centric, making it ill-equipped to address the unique cognitive and behavioural patterns of neurodivergent people. Existing studies, often designed and interpreted through a neurotypical lens, fail to capture the diversity of neurodivergent experiences, further limiting its relevance and efficacy.

This critique can be applied to any form behavioural modification advocated within therapeutic practices, particularly for autistic individuals, as it risks reinforcing internalised ableism and promoting masking by framing natural responses as problematic. Instead, the focus should shift towards societal change that values and supports neurodivergent ways of being, enabling acceptance and understanding over conformity.

Cognitive dissonance 💬

Cognitive dissonance occurs when a person holds two conflicting beliefs or engages in behaviour that contradicts their beliefs, resulting in psychological discomfort and stress. This internal tension often prompts a drive to reduce inconsistency through justification, minimisation, or change of one of the beliefs or actions. For neurodivergent individuals, this tension may be heightened by navigating environments that demand masking or adhering to neurotypical norms, which are at odds with their authentic self. For example, an autistic person may be compelled to suppress natural forms of communication, such as stimming, to fit society expectations of appropriate behaviour in public spaces, creating a state of cognitive dissonance and significant mental strain.

Colour vision deficiency 💬

Colour vision deficiency (CVD), or colour blindness, refers to conditions affecting the ability to perceive colours due to variations in the retina's cone cells. It ranges from mild difficulty distinguishing colours like red and green to severe limitations in the colour spectrum. CVD is slightly more common among autistic people than non-autistics, who may also experience heightened or reduced sensitivity to particular colours as part of their sensory processing differences. Adaptive strategies and inclusive design in environments and digital media can support people with CVD.

Communication books and passports 👥 🗨

These are personalised tools designed to help those with communication differences express their needs, preferences, and important information in settings like healthcare, education, or daily life. Communication books often include pictures, symbols, or written words, while passports summarise essential details like likes, dislikes, triggers, and support strategies.

These tools enable professionals and carers to tailor interactions, minimise misunderstandings, and respect the individual's autonomy. For example, a communication passport can help healthcare staff avoid sensory triggers, while a communication book allows teachers to adapt their methods. By facilitating clear and respectful exchanges, these resources empower individuals to have their voices heard and understood.

Communication regulation partner 👥 🗨

A communication regulation partner (CRP) is someone who facilitates and supports the communicative interactions of others, tailoring their approach to suit unique communication styles, including those of non-speaking or minimally speaking individuals. Integral to producing an inclusive communicative environment, CRPs must be keenly in tune with the person's body language to distinguish between purposeful movements and involuntary impulses. They should be trained in regulation techniques to assist when the individual becomes dysregulated, promoting a sense of calm and understanding.

CRPs build deep, trust-based relationships, often resembling familial bonds, to provide genuine support. With patience, kindness, and adaptability, they encourage individuals to realise their potential while challenging societal norms around communication. CRPs advocate for diverse, respectful methods that celebrate neurodivergent needs.

IN MY OWN WORDS: BEN BREAUX

Communication Regulation Partners (CRPs) help facilitate my communication through transcribing what I spell out on a letter board and knowing how to interpret what I say with my iPad.

Like any other job, my new CRPs need to undergo rigorous training. This includes learning how to use the Letterboard – my preferred method of communication – specifically with regards to positioning and reading my movements. Once our relationship is built, we can achieve "fluency," meaning we feel comfortable being alone together and can communicate with ease. The training period varies from CRP to CRP depending on a variety of factors, such as their prior experience and personality. I tend to warm up quickly to confident, smart people. If they are anxious, it makes me anxious, which can become a never ending cycle and thus we don't get work done. I also like hardcore people since they match my work ethic.

In addition to Letterboarding (or "Spelling"), I use my iPad for communicating basic needs. However, not everything I say with my iPad is clear to an outside perspective without a translator to help. For example, I tap "sea animals" on my iPad when I'm tired. This is a habit that stems from my childhood. When my family would go on trips, me and my sister would bring something from home for comfort and to help us sleep in new environments. My choice was a mini aquarium, which I still have to this day. Thus sparked the sea creatures on my iPad. Not everyone knows this story, so they may assume I am hitting random buttons with little reason. This is where my CRPs come in; they might help explain this, among other behaviors, to those who don't know or understand me. CRPs make sure I am heard by everyone and, fulfilling the "regulation" part of their title, make sure I am comfortable.

Certain stimuli, such as loud noises and bright lights, inhibit my enjoyment of various activities. My team of CRPs are there to help during these tough times by giving me assurance, fidget toys, snacks, and granting me space, if needed, to self-regulate. They also help keep me on track with my various responsibilities, such as my job as a blog writer as well as my delivery job. In addition, they help me with my schooling as I attempt to gain my full academic high school diploma. This includes reading the lessons out loud and going over notes with me, acting almost as my teacher.

My CRPs are near and dear to me, and I don't know what I would do without them.

Communication through behaviour

The concept of 'communication through behaviour' highlights how autistic and neurodivergent individuals may use actions, alone or alongside words, to express needs, feelings, or responses to their environment. This form of communication is often misunderstood or pathologised by observers, such as labelling someone with 'challenging behaviour' when, in fact, the individual is signalling distress or discomfort. This highlights the importance of recognising that all behaviour has communicative intent, especially for those who might struggle with traditional forms of communication. Understanding behaviour as a form of communication shifts the focus from attempting to 'fix' the behaviour to addressing the underlying needs or causes.

IN MY OWN WORDS: BEN BREAUX

The communication in my behavior isn't always clear. I often feel overwhelmed with the constant stimuli around me. This can manifest in my body doing things that may be confusing to others such as dumping my food or drinks. This is an example of unintentional body movements. My apraxia makes my body feel not like my own. My dumping is aggravating to myself and often to others. They don't usually understand that it's against my wishes. Actions have to be purposeful movement to be communication.

It is frustrating to be so misunderstood. The more I do impulsive things the harder it is to stop. So people often think I want to be doing what I'm doing. But that could not be further from the truth. These impulses don't come from

> nowhere. Often I am in dysregulation before my body shows it. Everything in my world is energy, so when the energy is off, I get anxious. This anxiety builds in my body and I lose control of it (my body). Doing things I don't want it to do and increasing the stressful energy. What I need in these moments is compassion and for people to understand that I want to stop. How can I be expected to stop when everyone is treating me like an idiot?
>
> If people understood it is often anxiety or dysregulation that I am communicating and that my actions are not necessarily directly related to what I'm actually intending to be doing, then I – and what it happening – will make more sense.

Community spaces

Community spaces refer to physical or virtual environments designed to create social interaction, support, 'social capital,' and engagement within a community. For neurodivergent individuals, these spaces are vital as they provide inclusive, accessible environments that celebrate neurological differences. They act as safe havens for sharing experiences, spreading knowledge, and promoting mutual understanding.

Effective community spaces are adaptable to diverse sensory needs, communication styles, and social preferences, enabling equitable and authentic participation. When designed and led by neurodivergent individuals or allies, they are more likely to succeed, gain credibility, and advocate for neurodivergence acceptance. By prioritising acceptance and support over conformity and intervention, community spaces contribute significantly to the well-being and empowerment of neurodivergent individuals, promoting a more inclusive society.

Competency-based questions vs hypothetical-based questions

Competency-based questions and hypothetical-based questions represent two distinct approaches in assessing an individual's suitability for a role. Competency-based questions focus on past behaviour and experiences, asking for real-life examples that demonstrate skills and abilities. This approach highlights tangible evidence of capabilities, making it especially inclusive for neurodivergent individuals by showcasing their unique strengths and practical achievements.

In contrast, hypothetical-based questions pose theoretical scenarios, requiring candidates to speculate on how they might respond to future situations. This approach can unfairly disadvantage neurodivergent individuals who excel in concrete thinking but may struggle with abstract reasoning.

The choice between these approaches affects inclusivity in the selection processes, underscoring the importance of tailoring assessment methods to support diverse cognitive styles, thereby promoting a more inclusive and equitable workplace.

Complex PTSD 🗨 🌿 🚫

Complex post-traumatic stress disorder (C-PTSD) is a psychological phenomenon caused by prolonged exposure to traumatic stress, notably within contexts of captivity, manipulation, power imbalance, or entrapment, where escape appears futile. Unlike PTSD, which stems from singular incidents, C-PTSD develops through chronic trauma and is marked by feelings of worthlessness, distrust, and a distorted sense of self. Neurodivergent individuals are particularly vulnerable due to societal marginalisation and adverse experiences. Supporting individuals with C-PTSD requires empathetic, trauma-informed care that supports healing and challenges structures sustaining trauma.

Concealment 🚫

Concealment refers to the deliberate hiding of one's neurological identity due to fear of stigma, discrimination, or misunderstanding. This phenomenon is particularly prevalent among neurodivergent individuals, including those who are autistic or ADHD or who identify with other neurological differences that society may misinterpret, misunderstand, or devalue. Concealment can lead to significant psychological distress, including feelings of isolation, low self-esteem, and anxiety, as individuals suppress their natural behaviours to conform to neurotypical standards. While concealment might offer temporary protection from immediate societal judgement, it undermines the individual's authenticity and can hinder meaningful connections with others.

Courtesy stigma 🌿 🚫

Courtesy stigma, also known as associative stigma, encapsulates the prejudice and discrimination extended to individuals closely associated with neurodivergent persons. It highlights how stigma extends beyond individuals to affect their support networks, often leading to internalised stigma among family members or caregivers. This can harm mental health, causing feelings of shame, guilt, and isolation.

Courtesy stigma arises from misconceptions and societal biases against neurodivergence, demonstrating the far-reaching impact of prejudice. Addressing it requires evidence-based education, awareness, and efforts to challenge negative attitudes towards neurodivergence.

Cultural communication 👥

Cultural communication involves the exchange of information shaped by societal norms, values, and practices, including both speaking and non-speaking interactions. Within the framework of neurodiversity, cultural communication takes on added layers of complexity as it intersects with the diverse ways in which neurodivergent individuals perceive, process, and express information. Valuing these differences enables inclusivity and enriches cross-cultural dialogues. Recognising neurodivergent communication styles challenges narrow, monolithic views of culture, promoting empathy, adaptability, and a deeper appreciation of human diversity. Building mutual respect requires continuous learning and a commitment to understanding cultural and neurological differences.

Cultural competence 👥

Cultural competence is the ability to understand, value, and engage effectively with people from diverse backgrounds, incorporating knowledge of different cultural practices into behaviour and attitudes. In neurodiversity, it involves recognising how neurodivergence intersects with cultural identities, shaping experiences, communication, and needs. For example, a neurodivergent person from a high-context culture, where non-verbal cues are crucial, might find it challenging to interpret subtle social signals due to their preference for direct communication. Achieving cultural competence requires ongoing learning, reflection, and proactive efforts to support inclusivity. It enables environments where neurodivergent individuals from all cultures feel respected, valued, and understood, promoting equity and collaboration across neurological and cultural differences.

IN MY OWN WORDS: HAZEL LIM

Working with Chinese neurodivergent individuals and their families, who are immigrants and minorities in the UK, has underscored the importance of cultural competence for me. As a multilingual autism specialist of Malaysian Chinese heritage, I fully appreciate how deeply culture shapes beliefs and perceptions.

Local services, including schools and healthcare providers, often operate with limited cultural awareness of neurodiversity. This can lead to misinterpretations of behaviours exhibited by neurodivergent individuals, such as viewing traits of autism as rudeness or non-compliance. Through training sessions and open dialogues, I have worked to bridge understanding between service providers and the neurodivergent Chinese community. Cultural competence is vital not only for recognising different cultural norms but also for valuing how neurodivergence manifests across cultures.

In Chinese culture, there is a deep-seated stigma surrounding mental health, neurodiversity, and disabilities. Discussing these topics is often seen as taboo, bringing shame to the family and disrupting communal harmony. This cultural backdrop influences how neurodivergence is perceived and managed. Traditional values, deeply rooted in history, resist open discussions of personal challenges. Tackling this stigma requires patience, education, and sustained effort, as these misconceptions are deeply ingrained.

Cultural competence involves ongoing learning and adaptation. By applying it in my personal and professional life, I aim to foster a society that respects neurodiversity in all its forms. Recognising the cultural stigma within the Chinese community, I prioritise promoting cultural competence both within this community and among the wider population. This includes educating service providers about the unique challenges faced by Chinese neurodivergent individuals and encouraging culturally sensitive approaches. For example, understanding that a lack of eye contact is a common autistic trait, not a sign of disrespect, can enhance interactions.

Cultural competence extends beyond awareness to include actionable steps, such as translation services, culturally relevant resources, and training for support staff to respect cultural nuances. One success story I remember involved a local school that initially struggled to support a Chinese neurodivergent student due to cultural misunderstandings. Through multiple meetings and training workshops, the staff learned about the cultural context and specific needs of the student and why the parents were initially reluctant to discuss their child's difficulties. The school implemented changes such as providing information in Mandarin for the parents and adopting communication strategies aligned with the family's cultural expectations. The result was a more supportive and understanding environment for the student, who subsequently thrived both academically and socially. Every life matters.

Chinese culture, with its deeply rooted values passed through generations, presents unique challenges in addressing stigma. However, by educating service providers and adopting culturally sensitive practices, we can create inclusive environments. This work involves recognising cultural nuances, accommodating differences, and enabling respect.

In conclusion, cultural competence is essential for building inclusive environments where neurodivergent individuals from all backgrounds can be accepted and thrive. By continuously learning and adapting, we can break down barriers, improve understanding, and create a society that truly values neurodiversity. Through my efforts, I hope to contribute to a broader acceptance of cultural differences, ensuring that everyone is heard, understood, and supported.

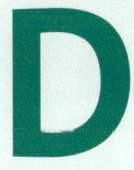

D

Deadnaming 🚫

Deadnaming is the harmful act of using a transgender or gender-diverse person's former name without consent after they have chosen a name that aligns with their gender identity. This invalidates their identity, causing distress, dysphoria, and alienation. In the neurodivergent community, where gender diversity is common, addressing deadnaming is essential. Respecting chosen names affirms identity, supports well-being, and enables inclusive environments that prioritise empathy, understanding, and acceptance.

Dedicated interests

Dedicated interests, often associated with autistic individuals, represent a deep and enduring engagement with specific topics or activities. Preferred over 'special interests,' this term emphasises the meaningful role these passions play in an individual's life. They are a source of joy, identity, and personal growth, offering cognitive, emotional, and social benefits.

Despite their value, dedicated interests are sometimes stigmatised as obsessive or unusual, leading some to view them as behaviours that need to be suppressed. This stigma increases the risk of harmful behavioural modification approaches aimed at curbing these interests, which can damage self-esteem and well-being and lead to trauma. Such responses run contrary to ethical approaches that advocate leaning into these interests and leveraging them as strengths.

Default mode network of the brain

The brain's default mode network (DMN) is a network of brain regions active during rest or passive states, facilitating self-reflection, daydreaming, memory recall, and introspection. For example, while walking, a wandering mind might revisit past conversations or plan future events. The DMN connects memories, insights, and future possibilities, enabling mental rehearsal and reframing of experiences. This process is essential for building self-understanding, planning, and a coherent sense of identity.

Deflective masking 💬 👥

Deflective masking refers to when an autistic person deflects attention from their own autistic identity – in an effort to conceal or mask their identity – by shifting focus onto another individual, often another autistic person. For example, an autistic parent may conceal their own neurodivergent traits by highlighting or overemphasising their child's autistic characteristics, thus avoiding scrutiny of their own identity. This strategy of masking serves as a way to navigate social situations by diverting attention away from themselves, often to evade judgement, misunderstanding, or stigmatisation. Deflective masking can be mentally exhausting and may lead to a disconnection from one's authentic self.

Demand avoidance 💬

Demand avoidance, often linked to autism, reflects an often anxiety-driven need for autonomy and control over one's environment. It arises from a mismatch between external demands and an individual's neurological needs, leading to anxiety, frustration, and protective responses. It is not wilfulness or defiance but a conscious and unconscious protective psychological reaction to overwhelming demands influenced by sensory sensitivities, executive functioning differences, and the need for predictability.

Excessive demands, or 'demand overload,' can cause stress responses like meltdowns or shutdowns, with severe mental health repercussions if escape or negotiation is not possible. Supporting autistic individuals involves adapting environments, respecting autonomy, and reducing demands to prevent harm and promote well-being. This shift prioritises understanding and acceptance over change, safeguarding mental and emotional health.

IN MY OWN WORDS: LYRIC RIVERA

Demand Avoidance is a trait that occurs along a continuum and can affect people of all ages. It is characterized by a natural inclination to resist or avoid others' demands, requests, or expectations. It can be a normal response to feeling overwhelmed, stressed, or frustrated.

Most people experience demand avoidance from time to time, and it can manifest in various ways, such as procrastination, excuse-making, avoiding responsibility, and passive-aggressive behavior.

This avoidance can range from typical demand avoidance (that most people experience from time to time) with little to no disruption to one's daily life, to more extreme forms of Demand Avoidance that are clinically diagnosable (as with Pathological Demand Avoidance or PDA, also known as Persistent Drive for Autonomy – which I, as a PDAer, like better).

Many individuals with PDA also meet the criteria for Autism. But it's essential to note that Demand Avoidance is not exclusive to Autism, and individuals who are not Autistic can also exhibit Demand Avoidance behaviors. However, the co-occurrence of Demand Avoidance and Autism is significant, and understanding this relationship can help with more effective support and accommodations for Autistic People who fit the PDA profile.

PDAers need far more autonomy than most people.

For PDAers, demands can pose much bigger problems than those with "average" demand tolerance.

In our high-demand society, PDA can be disruptive and even debilitating, especially when those of us who have increased levels of Demand Avoidance find ourselves in high-demand situations.

For us, Demand Avoidance can significantly affect daily functioning, relationships, and social interactions.

PDAers are often misunderstood and mislabeled as "non-compliant" or "oppositional," but the amount of autonomy each person needs to succeed is a legitimate aspect of our identities.

When demands are placed on individuals with more intense presentations of Demand Avoidance, we might experience feelings of suffocation or entrapment, intense anxiety or panic, and an overwhelming need to escape or control the situation.

When someone demands or expects something of me, I can feel trapped in a dangerous situation (or like I am being forced into something life-threatening).

My threat response is triggered even if I logically know better. My anxiety spikes, and I might shut down or lash out.

Sometimes, my reaction can be subtle.

I might be able to keep all my anguish and frustration to myself (so this avoidance goes unnoticed by those around me). Other times, when I cannot contain it, it spills over.

I've learned to recognize the signs – the feeling of suffocation and the intense need to escape or control the situation.

Demands from others can feel like threats, triggering a Demand Avoidant Person's fight-or-flight response.

My brain is constantly on high alert, awaiting subsequent demands or expectations.

When a demand comes, I feel like I'm walking on eggshells, trying not to trigger a meltdown, shutdown, or another type of overload because, at any minute, my world could come crashing down around me (or at least I could be triggered into feeling like it is).

I often feel like I'm fighting against my own brain, trying to find ways to cope, but I've also learned to advocate for myself and to communicate my needs and boundaries.

When people respect my boundaries, a weight lifts off my shoulders.

I wish more people understood what life as a PDAer is like. It's not about being "difficult" or "oppositional"; it's just how my brain works.

Instead, it's an experience that requires understanding, empathy, and compassion.

Demand sensitivity

Demand sensitivity describes the experience of autistic individuals whose mental and emotional resources, or 'spoons,' are quickly depleted when responding to external demands. The sensitivity to everyday pressures, expectations, and other demands intensifies as the person is left with fewer spoons, making each subsequent demand even more taxing and challenging to navigate. Acknowledging demand sensitivity shifts the focus towards creating environments that minimise undue stress and maximise autonomy and well-being, enabling a society that appreciates and supports neurodivergent ways of engaging with the world.

Depression

Depression is a complex mental health condition that profoundly affects mood, energy levels, well-being, and overall life perspective. While it can impact anyone, neurodivergent individuals, in particular autistic people, often experience depression due to lifelong stigma, discrimination, and the stress of navigating a world designed for neurotypicals. This chronic strain increases their vulnerability to depression, which can be seen as a rational response to trauma and exclusion rather than an irrational pathology.

Reducing depression in neurodivergent populations requires addressing societal attitudes, enabling inclusivity, and preventing internalised ableism. Autistic-led mental health support, such as therapy and groups led by autistic professionals, offers empathetic, tailored care grounded in shared experience and understanding.

Diagnosis

Traditionally, a diagnosis denotes the identification of a condition, usually with negative connotations, suggesting something 'abnormal,' which produces symptoms that are identified and enable a diagnosis. This medicalised framework contrasts with the view that neurological differences are natural variations, not deficits. While self-identification as autistic is empowering and often aligns with neurodiversity, a formal diagnosis is often necessary for accessing support and services in the current socio-medical system.

This creates tension between the aspiration for community-based recognition ('autistic identification') and the practical advantages of formal diagnosis. A future that acknowledges neurodivergent identities without medicalisation represents an aspirational shift. Such a framework would prioritise acceptance and support based on self-identified needs rather than medical labels. This transition is a crucial step towards a society that values and supports neurological differences beyond a medical context, moving closer to 'autopia.'

Diagnostic overshadowing 🚫

Diagnostic overshadowing occurs when a primary diagnosis, such as autism, causes other health concerns to be overlooked or underestimated. Healthcare professionals may attribute all health issues exclusively to an autism diagnosis, neglecting other potential underlying health conditions such as mental health issues and physical ailments. For example, trauma symptoms might be dismissed as part of autism, or severe depression misinterpreted as an intrinsic autistic trait.

This phenomenon not only impedes accurate medical assessment and treatment but also reinforces the stigma, contributing to a cycle of misunderstanding and neglect of neurodivergent individuals' complex needs. Addressing diagnostic overshadowing requires a holistic healthcare approach that values the full spectrum of an individual's health, ensuring all aspects of their well-being are recognised and treated.

Dialectical behaviour therapy 🏷️ 🚫

Dialectical behaviour therapy (DBT) is a cognitive-behavioural therapy originally developed for borderline personality disorder but has been adapted for broader use. It focuses on emotional regulation, mindfulness, and balancing acceptance with change. The approach is 'dialectical,' emphasising the balance between acceptance and change.

However, DBT faces criticism, particularly from trauma survivors and neurodivergent individuals, for its pathologising language and emphasis on behavioural change over addressing systemic issues like trauma and marginalisation. Emotional responses stemming from abuse or adverse experiences can be dismissed as 'problem behaviours,' leaving clients feeling invalidated or retraumatised. For autistic individuals, DBT may feel coercive, prioritising conformity to neurotypical norms over respecting neurodivergent ways of being. Its frameworks may also fail to account for sensory sensitivities or the need for predictability.

Therefore, while DBT may offers some valuable strategies, its effectiveness depends on adaptations that respect neurodivergent identities, validate lived experiences, and integrate trauma-informed care to ensure support is empowering and inclusive.

Digital rejection sensitivity dysphoria 💬 🌿

Digital rejection sensitivity dysphoria (digital RSD) is an extension of rejection sensitivity dysphoria, manifesting specifically in digital and online interactions. Like RSD, digital RSD is characterised by intense reactions to perceived or real rejection; however, it is uniquely heightened in online contexts such as social media, emails, or messaging apps. The immediacy and ambiguity of digital communication can amplify distress, as those with digital RSD may misinterpret delayed responses, lack of 'likes' or engagement, or seemingly neutral messages as signs of rejection or criticism.

This can lead to deep feelings of anxiety, sadness, or anger, often stemming from past experiences of exclusion or rejection magnified by the inherently impersonal nature of digital communication. People experiencing digital RSD may engage in hyper-vigilance, people-pleasing, or avoidant behaviours online to minimise perceived threats of rejection, sometimes resulting in emotional exhaustion or withdrawal from digital spaces.

Digital twinning 🏷️ 🏢

Digital twinning refers to the creation of a digital replica of a physical entity or system. This enables real-time monitoring, simulation, and analysis, providing a platform for exploring potential support strategies and environments. For instance, an autistic student overwhelmed by noise and visual stimuli in a traditional classroom could benefit from a digital twin of the learning space. This virtual replica could adjust lighting, noise, and layout to optimise the student's sensory and learning styles. Educators could experiment with setups to find the most supportive environment.

Digital twinning offers opportunities for individualised educational tools, adaptive learning environments, and personalised healthcare that are neurodivergent-affirming. However, privacy, data security, and surveillance risks must be addressed to ensure these technologies enhance rather than compromise neurodivergent autonomy and well-being.

Direct questions

Direct questions is a communication strategy where questions are posed in a straightforward, unambiguous manner. This approach is often particularly beneficial for autistic people, who may find implicit cues, inferred meanings, or rhetorical questions challenging to navigate. Direct questioning respects neurodivergent communication styles, promoting clarity and reducing the cognitive load associated with deciphering vague or implied content. The practice underscores the importance of understanding and respecting diverse communication needs, advocating for adjustments in conversational norms to boost inclusivity.

Disability Discrimination Act 1995

The Disability Discrimination Act represents a cornerstone in UK legislation, aimed at ending the discrimination that many disabled people face. Enacted in 1995 and later superseded by the Equality Act 2010, the Act made it unlawful to discriminate against individuals with disabilities in connection with employment, the provision of goods and services, education, and transport. However, while the Act marked a significant step forward in promoting equality, its implementation has faced challenges. This includes the view that legal protections alone are insufficient without robust enforcement and societal change and that legislation must evolve to reflect a more nuanced understanding of disability and neurodiversity.

Disability Living Allowance

Disability Living Allowance (DLA) is a UK government-funded benefit aimed at providing financial support to individuals with disabilities, acknowledging the additional expenses incurred due to disability. While DLA is specific to children in the UK, its adult counterpart has transitioned to Personal Independence Payment (PIP), reflecting ongoing welfare reforms. This transition has sparked debate about whether the new system adequately meets the needs of disabled people, with some arguing that it has led to stricter assessments and reduced entitlements for many, in turn, potentially compromising the well-being and independence of individuals with disabilities.

Other countries have similar initiatives. In the US, Social Security Disability Insurance (SSDI) supports disabled individuals with sufficient work history, while Supplemental Security Income (SSI) aids those in financial need. Australia's Disability Support Pension (DSP) assists those unable to work due to physical, intellectual, or mental health problems.

These benefits, while essential, face criticism over their accessibility, adequacy, and the complexity of their application processes, which can hinder people in genuine need accessing the support. The requirement for extensive documentation and proof of disability can be particularly challenging for individuals with fluctuating or less visible disabilities, leading to potential underrepresentation and support gaps. Critics also argue the financial assistance is insufficient to meet the additional living costs faced by disabled individuals, leaving many vulnerable.

Disclosure

Disclosure refers to the act of revealing one's neurodivergent identities, such as being autistic, dyslexic, or ADHD, in various social, educational, or employment settings. This process is deeply personal and carries potential risks and benefits. On one hand, disclosure can lead to greater understanding, support, adaptations and accommodations, facilitating a more inclusive environment that respects neurodivergent ways of being. However, it may also expose individuals to stigma, discrimination, and misunderstanding, highlighting the precarious balance between seeking support and risking marginalisation. The decision to disclose is influenced by numerous factors, including the anticipated response, the importance of obtaining support, and personal comfort with one's neurodivergent identity. This highlights the importance of creating a society where disclosure is always likely to be safe and supportive experience, where individuals feel accepted and valued for their unique contributions, irrespective of neurotype.

IN MY OWN WORDS: JOAN LAPLANA

I always knew that I was different. As I was growing up, I got used to being "the odd one." But I never thought I was autistic.

Everything changed when my son was a toddler and the health visitor suggested that he might be autistic. We started the process to gain a

diagnosis, but we stopped at the last hurdle because we didn't want to put a label to our son. But when he was a teenager, we finally went through with all the process and our son was diagnosed with Asperger's syndrome. It was then when my ex-wife dropped the bomb to me: "if our son is autistic, you are autistic too." The penny dropped. That started a journey where after the initial shame due my unconscious bias I started to explore the possibility more.

I did not tell anyone as I was afraid of the stigma. I learnt to comply. Everything changed when Sally, one of my nurses, came and asked me for advice and help. Sally was autistic and wanted to know if I knew of any support networks that could help her. I started to look for answers, but I couldn't find one. I was shocked. That was the moment I knew I wanted to do something about it.

I admired Sally. She was not hiding and was openly autistic at work in the hope that it will challenge stereotypes and gradually improve the working lives of autistic nurses. I wasn't as brave as her, and at that point, I kept my autism journey secret until then. That day I decided to disclose my autistic identity publicly and try to make things easy for autistic nurses. I learnt the hard way.

Being autistic in nursing has its challenges. I have burned out due to the demands of nursing, the environment, the unrelenting workload. But somehow, I have always managed to bounce back. It is not made easier when your colleagues (across all grades) refuse to believe your diagnosis or make comments such as "you don't look autistic" or "you must be high functioning." I want my strengths to be seen and valued. I want to be viewed as an individual who is more than a diagnosis.

Discrimination 🚫

Discrimination is the unjust and prejudicial treatment of individuals based on distinct characteristics, such as neurodivergence, race, gender, or disability. Discrimination is a pivotal issue among neurodivergent individuals given that they often face barriers that inhibit full and equitable participation in society. Such discrimination arises from myriad sources, including professionals in healthcare, education, and employers, alongside systemic issues within organisations such as workplaces, educational institutions, and public services. Discrimination not only impacts individual well-being and opportunities but also leads to and perpetuates stigma and exclusion, undermining the principles of equality and diversity. The journey towards eradicating discrimination demands rigorous enforcement of existing laws, alongside a cultural transformation that champions diversity and equality at every level.

IN MY OWN WORDS: HAZEL LIM

Autism means I see, smell, taste, touch, and listen to the world differently. As a neurodivergent individual, my journey through life involves managing compulsive behaviours, social challenges, and sensory sensitivities, as well as confronting societal attitudes and barriers to acceptance. These daily navigations are integral to my experience and shape how I interact with the world around me.

Within the Chinese community, the journey for autistic individuals and their families is compounded by layers of discrimination. Beyond the universal challenges faced by all neurodivergent individuals, such as health disparities and societal biases, there are additional hurdles rooted in cultural beliefs and misunderstandings. These unique obstacles make it even more difficult for us to find acceptance and understanding within our own cultural context.

For Chinese immigrants living in the UK, the intersectionality of their immigrant status and neurodivergence compounds the challenges they face. In addition to navigating the complexities of relocation, language barriers, and cultural adjustment, they must also confront the stigma surrounding neurodiversity within both their own community and broader society. This results in more than double discrimination, leading to profound isolation and exclusion.

Many Chinese families living in the UK, fearing the repercussions of this stigma, may choose to conceal their child's condition and limit social interactions. This isolation is compounded by the perception of autism as contagious or shameful, leading to further ostracisation within immigrant communities.

Consider, for example, a Chinese family immigrating to the UK with an autistic child. Already grappling with the challenges of adapting to a new country, they now face the added burden of navigating the stigma surrounding autism. Language barriers further complicate their access to information and support services, leaving them doubly marginalized and struggling to access vital resources.

Faced with a lack of understanding and support, these families may find themselves isolated within their own community, unable to seek the assistance they desperately need. The fear of being labelled as "different" or "less than" further exacerbates their sense of alienation, leaving them feeling like outsiders in a society that fails to recognise their unique strengths and contributions.

In my own journey as an autistic individual, I have encountered firsthand the impact of discrimination and misunderstanding. It often involves layers of dignity and vulnerability. From exclusion in social settings to subtle biases in academic and professional environments, the barriers to acceptance are pervasive.

However, rather than being defined by these challenges, I have chosen to embrace my neurodivergence as a strength. Living like an open book, I am transparent about my differences and position myself as a role model. By advocating for greater awareness and understanding, I have not only received recognition and awards in my professional capacity but, more importantly, sparked conversations and produced empathy. Despite these efforts, I still face discrimination on many occasions, and it is something that should not be underestimated – it hurts.

Dissociative identity disorder

Formerly known as multiple personality disorder, dissociative identity disorder (DID) is a complex psychological condition characterised by the presence of two or more distinct identity or personality states that control an individual's behaviour at different times. These identities, each with their unique patterns of perceiving and interacting with the world, emerge as a response to severe trauma, often during early childhood. DID challenges traditional notions of a singular, cohesive identity, proposing instead that the mind can compartmentalise experiences, particularly traumatic ones, to protect the individual. Support focuses on integrating these identities into a cohesive self and addressing the underlying trauma.

Double empathy problem

The double empathy problem, introduced by Dr Damian Milton, challenges traditional views of autism and social interaction. This theory posits that the communication difficulties between autistic and non-autistic individuals are bidirectional rather than inherently stemming from autistic people. Both groups struggle to understand and empathise with each other due to differing ways of processing and interpreting social cues. Autistic individuals often communicate effectively within their neurotype, as do non-autistic people. However, cross-neurotype interactions reveal mismatched communication styles, such as an autistic person missing subtle facial expressions or a non-autistic person misinterpreting directness as rudeness. This theory emphasises the need for mutual understanding and adaptation, urging society to recognise and value diverse communication styles.

Dyscalculia

Dyscalculia is a neurological difference affecting how people understand and process number-based concepts, including quantities, symbols, and patterns. It goes beyond difficulty with arithmetic and affects around 3–7% of the population. Dyscalculia is linked to differences in brain structure, particularly in the parietal lobe, which is crucial for numerical processing.

For example, a dyscalculic individual might struggle with concepts like 'greater than' or 'less than,' even if they can read numbers correctly. When comparing 7 and 12, they may find it difficult to recognise that 12 is larger. Similarly, they might have trouble telling the time on an analogue clock, finding it challenging to interpret the positions of the hands as specific numbers or intervals.

Dysgraphia

Dysgraphia is a neurological difference affecting the ability to produce written language. It is lifelong, present from birth, and does not diminish over time. Dysgraphia often becomes apparent in childhood through challenges such as poor spelling, inconsistent letter sizes, poor spatial planning of words, and difficulty organising thoughts in writing. These difficulties can become more pronounced in adulthood due to increased writing demands in academic or professional settings.

There are various forms of dysgraphia, such as motor dysgraphia, which is linked to fine motor skill difficulties, and phonological dysgraphia, which affects spelling irregular or unfamiliar words like 'knight' or 'yacht'. Despite these challenges, dysgraphia is not linked to intelligence; rather, it reflects a divergence in how the brain processes writing tasks.

Dyskinesia

Dyskinesia is characterised by involuntary, erratic muscle movements that can be challenging due to their unpredictability and impact on day-to-day activities or interactions. It is often a side effect of treatments like antipsychotics or Parkinson's medications. Dyskinesia includes various movement disorders, such as paroxysmal kinesigenic dyskinesia, a rare condition where sudden voluntary movements, like standing or walking, trigger brief episodes of involuntary movements lasting seconds to minutes. Tardive dyskinesia is another form, involving repetitive, involuntary movements of the face and tongue, often developing after a few months of medication use and sometimes persisting even after the drug is stopped.

Dyslexia

Dyslexia is a neurological difference that relates to how a person processes written language. It is often characterised by difficulties with reading, spelling, and writing, although dyslexic individuals often excel in other areas, particularly in creative, innovative, and problem-solving domains often because of their ability to see the 'big picture' in a given scenario. However, dyslexia varies in its presentation; not all individuals will experience the same difficulties or strengths.

Dyslexia is hereditary, so a child has a 40–60% chance of being dyslexic if one parent is dyslexic, rising to 60–80% if both parents are dyslexic. Dyslexia is unrelated to intelligence and represents a distinct cognitive profile within neurodivergence. It is not a deficit requiring a cure but a unique way of processing information that can be advantageous when supported and nurtured.

Dyspraxia

Dyspraxia, sometimes referred to as developmental coordination disorder (DCD), is a form of neurodivergence that affects motor planning – the brain's ability to organise and carry out coordinated muscle movements. It can impact both gross motor skills, such as coordination, balance, running, jumping, or navigating stairs, and fine motor skills, making tasks like writing, fastening buttons, or catching a ball more challenging. The degree and specific areas affected can vary between individuals, resulting in differing levels of support needs.

Dyspraxics often face challenges with organisation, planning, time management, and attention. Around 5–6% of people are dyspraxic, with males more frequently diagnosed. Support strategies include breaking tasks into steps and using tools like speech-to-text software, ergonomic keyboards, or visual timers. Personalised approaches that emphasise strengths are essential for building confidence and independence.

Dysregulation

Dysregulation describes a state where an individual's sensory, emotional, or behavioural responses are significantly unbalanced, often seen when environments and demands overwhelm an individual's capacity to self-manage. For many neurodivergent individuals, including autistic people, it is a natural reaction to overwhelming stimuli or demands that exceed their current capacity to cope.

Dysregulation can manifest as intense emotions, sensory overload, or an apparent loss of control. These are not behavioural 'problems' but authentic responses to unmet sensory or emotional needs, often worsened by environments poorly suited to neurodivergent ways of processing. Creating inclusive, safe spaces that support self-regulation is essential for helping individuals regain balance.

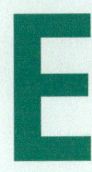

Eating disorders 🌿 🚫

Eating disorders encompass complex behaviours around food, body image, and eating, often shaped by social, cultural, and psychological factors. Sadly, society often misinterprets these as simple issues of diet or lifestyle.

For neurodivergent individuals, eating challenges may arise from sensory sensitivities or anxieties about routine. Autistic individuals, for example, might struggle with textures, flavours, or environmental factors that significantly affect their eating habits. Conditions like avoidant/restrictive food intake disorder (ARFID), which involves extreme food selectivity, can be common among autistic people, as it often stems from sensory aversions or the need for predictability in food choices. This is an example of how, for neurodivergent people, traditional understandings of 'eating disorders' may not fully apply, as their experiences are often shaped by factors beyond societal pressures of body image, such as sensory processing challenges or the need for consistency in food.

Autistic individuals are at additional risk of eating challenges due to the stigma and discrimination they may face, and especially if they are experiencing poor mental health. Alexithymia – difficulty recognising emotions – can worsen this by making food a tool for managing distress, even without a clear awareness of hunger.

Therapeutic approaches should adopt a neurodivergent-affirming perspective. Terms like 'eating challenges' or 'eating difficulties' are preferable to 'eating disorders,' as they avoid pathologising neurodivergent experiences.

IN MY OWN WORDS: GINNY GRANT

I have struggled with various forms of an eating disorder for many years. A poor body image arose from my high school years as a gymnast, where my physique was on show in a skimpy leotard at weekly competitions. Having a somewhat curvy, more athletic build than the average gymnast in my club,

DOI: 10.4324/9781003477297-5

I quickly recognised that I did not belong and put even more pressure upon myself to perform at a very high – impeccable – standard. At a deeper level, I recognise that my efforts as a young person to try to control my body shape, through dietary restriction and excessive exercise, were tied closely to my efforts to feel accepted more generally.

Much later, in my 30s, a restrictive eating disorder, identified as EDNOS (eating disorder – not otherwise specified), emerged, where I tracked nutritional intake, physical activity, and weight loss in an obsessive manner. Every morsel, every sip, every gram, every step went into the app on my phone. The app became as important to me as a deeply personal journal. It was my way of instilling control in a world that was all too often highly unpredictable, in a family situation with two neurodivergent children that diverged from the norm. The result: rapid, significant weight loss and numerous markers, and experiences, of ill health. With the support of my medical team and my loving family and friends, I came through the other side of this cruel eating disorder, only to relapse several years later at a time of peak stress. This time my medical team was ready for me, understood precisely how this eating disorder affected me, and was quick to intervene before it became as serious as the previous time.

Sometimes I ask myself whether I will ever fully recover from this cruel eating disorder. I want to say, 'of course I will,' for me, but I know now that my brain is wired a certain way, I am highly vulnerable to environmental factors and old habits die hard. In the meantime, I lean on my support team unapologetically, because I choose to live.

Echolalia

Echolalia is the automatic repetition of full words and phrases as well as parts of words or phrases. It can also include mimicking sounds, music, or even non-speaking sounds like environmental noises. It can occur immediately (immediate echolalia) or after a delay (delayed echolalia).

Echolalia serves many purposes, such as supporting language development, processing information, reducing anxiety, expressing emotions or needs, self-regulation, and providing a safe way to communicate. However, it is often stigmatised by society as problematic or meaningless repetition, when, in fact, it is a valid and useful form of communication.

Education Act 1996 ⚖️ 🏢

The Education Act 1996 is a cornerstone of educational legislation in England and Wales, offering a detailed framework for the operation of schools and the responsibilities of local authorities, particularly in relation to children with special educational needs and disabilities (SEND). Since its introduction, the Act has undergone several updates to adapt to the evolving educational landscape.

One of its enduring strengths lies in its commitment to recognising and supporting the diverse needs of learners, including neurodivergent students. The Act obliges local authorities to identify and assess children with SEND, promote inclusivity, and provide tailored support. However, it has faced criticism for insufficiently addressing the nuanced needs of neurodivergent learners. Processes can be rigid, causing delays in accessing necessary resources or adjustments. While it remains vital, ongoing reforms are needed to enhance flexibility and inclusivity.

Education, Health, and Care Plans ⚖️ 🛡️ 🏢

An Education, Health and Care Plan (EHCP) is a legally binding document in the United Kingdom designed to provide support for children and young people up to the age of 25 who have special educational needs (SEN). An EHCP outlines a person's educational, health, and social care needs and specifies the additional support required to meet those needs in educational settings. Crucially, EHCPs are not limited to academic challenges but also encompass social and emotional support needs, which makes them holistic in nature.

Despite the legal framework, many families face significant challenges in securing or implementing EHCPs due to issues such as miscommunication or funding cuts. If disagreements arise, there is an appeal process, and it is vital that parents and carers remain vigilant to ensure that the local authority provides the agreed support.

Educational advocacy ⚖️ 🛡️ 🏢

Educational advocacy ensures neurodivergent students receive equitable, inclusive education by addressing systemic barriers and securing necessary supports. Advocates work with schools to provide accommodations like personalised learning plans, sensory-friendly environments, and alternative communication methods. Advocacy empowers families and students by amplifying their voices, promoting self-advocacy, and challenging discrimination. It emphasises meeting the diverse needs of autistic learners by valuing their unique strengths and perspectives rather than forcing conformity to neurotypical standards.

Educational psychologists

Educational psychologists specialise in supporting the learning, behaviour, and emotional well-being of children and young people, particularly in educational settings. They collaborate with schools, families, and students to create supportive environments for neurodivergent learners. Their work often includes assessments to understand a student's cognitive and emotional profile, providing tailored recommendations. It is important that their approach does not reflect the medical model of disability, which can focus the psychologist on perceived deficits rather than strengths and can undervalue the social and systemic aspects that impact students' learning and well-being in educational contexts.

Ehlers-Danlos syndrome

Ehlers-Danlos syndrome (EDS) is a group of genetic conditions affecting connective tissues that support skin, joints, and blood vessels. Individuals with EDS often experience joint hypermobility, meaning their joints may be unusually flexible and prone to dislocation. Additionally, their skin can be highly elastic and fragile, bruising easily and taking longer to heal. There are multiple subtypes of EDS, each presenting different symptoms, but all result from genetic mutations that disrupt the production of collagen, a crucial component of connective tissue.

Hypermobile EDS (hEDS), a subtype of EDS, is frequently linked to neurodivergent individuals, in particular autistic people. This can bring challenges like chronic pain, proprioceptive difficulties, and dysautonomia, which affects heart rate, blood pressure, and digestion, causing symptoms such as dizziness and fainting.

Embodied identity

The term 'embodied identity' refers to the interconnectedness of a person's physical body and sense of self. It highlights how autistic and other neurodivergent individuals experience the world through their unique sensory, motor, and bodily experiences. For example, an autistic person might perceive a crowded room not just as a social space but as an overwhelming cascade of sounds, lights, and physical sensations that deeply influence their sense of belonging and self-expression. The concept rejects the idea of a disconnection between mind and body, promoting a more integrated view of identity, where bodily experiences are not separate from selfhood but intrinsic to navigating the world.

Emotional well-being

Emotional well-being is the experience of positive feelings such as happiness and contentment, alongside having the tools to understand, process, and express all emotions in ways that align with one's needs and values. It also encompasses resilience, self-awareness, emotional regulation, a sense of meaning and purpose, and the ability to build and maintain supportive relationships. However, traditional measures of emotional well-being often miss the mark for neurodivergent individuals. This is because neurodivergent individuals may experience emotions differently or face unique stressors related to social expectations, sensory sensitivities, and stigma. For instance, autistic individuals might experience heightened emotional reactions to environmental stimuli or empathic distress, while ADHD individuals may respond impulsively before fully processing a situation. Similarly, individuals with alexithymia may have difficulty identifying or describing their emotions, which can fundamentally alter how they experience and understand their emotional well-being. These examples highlight how emotional well-being for neurodivergent individuals may not always align with conventional expressions of emotional health.

Empathic distress

Empathic distress is the overwhelming emotional response experienced when witnessing another person's suffering, often to the extent that it impairs one's ability to provide meaningful support. This concept is particularly significant in the context of autistic experiences, as autistic people are frequently hyperempathic, feeling others' emotions with heightened intensity. Empathic distress goes beyond typical empathy; it creates a barrier where the emotional toll on the observer becomes so consuming that it limits their capacity to act constructively. For autistic people, sensory and emotional hypersensitivity can amplify this experience, leading to exhaustion, shutdowns, or a need to withdraw from emotionally charged situations.

Consider a scenario where an autistic teenager observes their parent in visible anguish after a family argument. They not only feel the weight of their parent's sorrow but also experience it as if it were their own, magnified through their heightened emotional sensitivity. The intensity of these feelings can be paralysing, leading the teenager to retreat to their room in tears, overwhelmed and unable to provide comfort. To outsiders, this might appear as selfishness or indifference, but in truth, it reflects the debilitating impact of empathic distress.

Empathy

Empathy is often misunderstood in relation to autistic people. A common myth is that autistic individuals lack empathy, but this is untrue and misleading. In fact, the majority of autistic people experience hyperempathy, meaning they may feel others' emotions more intensely than neurotypical individuals. For some, this may also mean that they sense emotions in others before those individuals are even aware of their own feelings. It is important to recognise that empathy can manifest differently depending on how one processes emotional and sensory information. Autistic people may struggle with identifying or expressing emotions in ways typically expected, but this should not be confused with a lack of empathy. Instead, they may demonstrate empathy in unique and profound ways.

Employee resource groups ⚖️ 🛡️ 🏢

Employee resource groups (ERGs) are groups formed and led by employees to voluntarily promote and support equity, diversity, and inclusion, especially for underrepresented communities, within their organisations. For neurodivergent employees, these groups can provide a platform to share experiences, seek support, and advocate for workplace adaptations and accommodations that meet divergent neurological needs. These groups can be a powerful tool for challenging traditional workplace norms, raising an understanding of neurodivergent strengths and enabling a culture of acceptance.

Employment advocacy ⚖️ 🛡️ 🏢

Employment advocacy supports and promotes the employment rights of neurodivergent individuals by addressing systemic barriers and biases that hinder access to meaningful employment. It emphasises the need for inclusive environments, necessary adaptations, and challenges discriminatory practices and unconscious biases that favour neurotypical candidates despite the skills and qualifications of neurodivergent individuals.

Advocates inform neurodivergent people about their employment rights and relevant laws and push to ensure that employers meet their legal obligations. Additionally, many workplaces have employee resource groups (ERGs), also known as equality, diversity, and inclusion (EDI) groups. These groups can be useful for enabling an inclusive culture and providing support.

IN MY OWN WORDS: JOAN LAPLANA

My career in nursing has been a roller coaster, filled with soaring highs and gut-wrenching lows. Depending on who you ask, I'm either a nightmare to work with or a genius. Some of my managers have likened me to Marmite – you either love me or hate me. Over the years, I've faced disciplinary panels four times and been dismissed three, yet I am also one of the most award-winning nurses in the NHS. How can these two extremes coexist? The answer is simple: the workplace culture.

Legally, I am considered disabled, but I don't believe the label fits. I see it differently: society and the environments we work in are what disable me.

That's why I've made it my mission to transform workplaces into neuroinclusive spaces where not just neurodivergent individuals, but everyone, can thrive.

One example of this mission in action is my work within the NHS and beyond, advocating for a shift in how neurodivergent people are perceived and supported. Managers often label individuals who don't conform as "troublemakers." Instead, I challenge them to ask a different question: could this person be neurodivergent? This simple shift in perspective can lead to a journey of understanding that benefits not only the individual but the entire team. I speak from experience because I've lived on both sides of the coin. I've been in hostile environments that led to trauma and dismissal, and I've worked in inclusive settings that celebrated my strengths and allowed me to thrive. I don't want others to endure the trauma I've faced or leave their success to chance. My goal is to ensure workplaces are designed to unlock the full potential of every individual.

When I disclose I am autistic, I'm often met with comments like, "But you don't look autistic – I can't see anything wrong with you." These remarks are frustrating because they reflect a fundamental misunderstanding. There is nothing "wrong" with me – I'm just different. Neurodivergent brains aren't disabled; they're wired differently.

Employers and managers must shift their focus away from what neurodivergent individuals struggle with and towards what they excel at. For example, in my work, I've advocated for practical changes such as flexible working hours, quiet workspaces, and tailored mentorship programmes. These adjustments don't just benefit neurodivergent individuals – they create a more inclusive, productive environment for everyone.

When I first realised I was autistic, I sought a support network where I could share my experiences and learn from others. To my surprise, there wasn't one. That sense of isolation spurred me to create the Neurodiverse Nurses UK network – a platform that now provides vital support, education, and pastoral care for neurodivergent nurses. It's one of my proudest achievements and a testament to what's possible when we build systems of support rather than perpetuate exclusion.

I've seen how employment advocacy can break down the stigma surrounding autism. When workplaces focus on unlocking the potential of neurodivergent individuals, they don't just help those individuals – they challenge and change societal narratives about autism. Personally, it's been a long journey of self-discovery. For years, I tried to fix what I thought was "wrong" with me. Therapy and reflection helped me realise there was nothing to fix. Today, I am proud to be autistic and fully comfortable in my own skin.

Employment advocacy is more than a strategy – it's a tool for transformation. By creating workplaces that celebrate neurodiversity, we not only remove stigma but also unleash the potential of people like me. When that happens, everyone wins.

Empowerment ⚖️ 🛡️

Empowerment involves autistic and other neurodivergent people reclaiming authorship over their narratives, controlling language, and enhancing self-advocacy skills. The journey from powerlessness to empowerment transforms perceptions and enhances mental well-being. This process enables personal growth, strengthens community connections, and reshapes self-concept. Empowerment also involves understanding lived experiences, challenging stereotypes, and improving quality of life in meaningful ways. It is about asserting autonomy, reclaiming agency, and countering internalised ableism. Achieving empowerment is easier when connected to the autistic community and more challenging if the individual has experienced significant stigma, ableism, and trauma. Despite these challenges, it is still possible to break away from these negative impacts through effective professional and community-based support and by benefiting from autistic-led mental health therapies.

IN MY OWN WORDS: HAZEL LIM

In the Chinese community, where hierarchy and authority hold significant sway, the belief persists that only professionals like doctors, teachers, or therapists can truly help neurodivergent children. Witnessing firsthand the struggles families face, particularly when confronted with lengthy waiting lists for services, I felt a profound sense of urgency to make a difference. Drawing from both my professional expertise as a multilingual autism specialist and my lived experience as a neurodivergent individual, I recognised the pressing need for meaningful change.

This realisation fuelled my determination to establish the non-profit organisation 'Chinese Autism CIC,' driven by a deep-seated desire to empower and build resilience within the Chinese neurodivergent community. My journey was shaped by what I've seen and heard, combined with an unwavering commitment to effect positive change. Through the organisation, I sought to challenge societal misconceptions, combat discrimination, and provide crucial support services.

At the heart of our mission lies empowerment – a concept I hold dear, rooted in my own experiences navigating the complexities of neurodivergence. By offering educational resources in both Chinese translations and English, we empower individuals and families to make informed decisions and challenge prevailing misconceptions about autism. Additionally, our emphasis on community-building and mutual support aims to counter the isolation often felt in the face of cultural stigma.

Advocacy and activism have been integral to our approach. Engaging with policymakers, healthcare professionals, and community leaders, I strive to amplify awareness and support for neurodivergent within the Chinese community. Through collaborative efforts and awareness campaigns, we endeavour to create a more inclusive and supportive society for all.

Recognising the unique challenges posed by language barriers and cultural norms, many passionate volunteers I've encountered along my journey have joined the team. We tailor our resources and support services to address these specific needs, ensuring that our empowerment efforts are accessible and relevant to those we serve. Ultimately, this empowers strength and belief in individuals to thrive despite the challenges they may encounter. Together, we are transforming stigma into strength and paving the way for a brighter future within the Chinese neurodiversity community.

Emulation 🗣 🌿 👥

For neurodivergent individuals, emulation refers to the adaptive process of imitating or mirroring neurotypical behaviours to navigate environments that do not support their neurological differences. This is closely related to the concept of masking or camouflaging, where autistic people adjust their natural behaviours to meet societal expectations, often at a significant emotional and mental health cost. Emulation is not a natural or preferred way of interacting for many neurodivergent people but is often used as a survival strategy in environments that are not neurodivergent-affirming. This can result in feelings of inauthenticity and increased anxiety, as it suppresses natural ways of being and interacting. Emulation highlights the importance of creating inclusive environments that allow neurodivergent individuals to express themselves authentically.

Enacted stigma 🌱 🚫

Enacted stigma refers to direct acts of discrimination and exclusion faced by marginalised groups. It ranges from subtle behaviours to overt actions that communicate prejudice, rejection, or mistreatment, such as being denied opportunities in education, employment, or healthcare. This stigma can severely impact mental health, increasing stress, anxiety, and social isolation.

A subtle example is when autistic individuals are excluded from social activities at work or school due to assumptions about their social preferences rather than being asked or included. A more blatant example is when an autistic student is denied school admission based on prejudiced beliefs about their perceived 'difficulty' or 'resource demands.'

For autistic people, enacted stigma often stems from misconceptions that their ways of thinking and behaving are 'deficient' rather than different. These harmful attitudes reinforce barriers to acceptance and inclusion. Addressing enacted stigma requires cultural and social change that promotes respect and values neurodivergent identities.

Energy accounting 💬 🌱

Energy accounting, also referred to as 'spoon theory' is the practice of managing and measuring one's physical, mental, and emotional energy. It recognises that neurodivergent people often have limited energy reserves (referred to metaphorically as 'spoons') and that different tasks and social interactions may deplete this energy more quickly than for neurotypical individuals.

Energy accounting helps autistic people prioritise essential tasks and make adjustments to conserve energy. For example, they might schedule quiet time between social activities to recharge or use noise-cancelling headphones to reduce sensory overload in busy environments.

However, if one's energy is depleted with more demands and tasks still ahead, it can lead to burnout, anxiety, distress, meltdowns, and shutdowns. Therefore, this concept is crucial in navigating a world designed with neurotypical expectations, as it allows individuals to engage in self-care, manage boundaries and personal limits, avoid burnout, and maintain a balance between activities and rest.

Empty phrases 💬 👥

Empty phrases, such as "How are you?" or "What's up?," are expressions primarily used to initiate or maintain social interaction without conveying meaningful content. Known as 'phatic language,' these phrases are common in non-autistic communication but can feel vague or confusing for many autistic people, often leading to awkwardness or anxiety.

Autistic individuals typically prefer clear, direct communication. Literal interpretations of these questions may prompt honest replies, sometimes surprising neurotypical counterparts. To navigate these exchanges, autistic people may rely on scripted responses like "I'm fine," but this can feel inauthentic and fail to create a genuine connection.

Entropy

The metaphor of entropy in relation to neurodiversity explores the complexity and unpredictability that arise from human cognitive and neurological diversity. Just as entropy in physics measures the degree of disorder within a system, neurodiversity suggests that neurological differences should be seen as natural variations rather than deviations from a norm. This metaphor can help us understand the value of diverse cognitive styles, emphasising that they contribute to innovation and problem-solving by introducing new perspectives and approaches. For example, neurodivergent thinkers like Alan Turing and Nikola Tesla used their unique cognitive patterns to revolutionise fields such as computing and electrical engineering. Their non-linear thinking styles were key to their breakthroughs, reflecting how embracing cognitive and neurological diversity (or 'entropy') can lead to societal advancements. Therefore, neurodivergent individuals, with their distinctive ways of perceiving and interacting with the world, add depth and richness to human experience, similar to how entropy adds complexity to physical systems.

Epilepsy

Epilepsy is a neurological condition that affects the brain's electrical activity, leading to recurrent, unprovoked seizures. These seizures result from abnormal bursts of electrical signals, which can affect various parts of the body depending on the seizure type. One in 26 people will develop epilepsy during their lifetime, making it one of the most common neurological conditions globally. About 70% of people with epilepsy could live seizure-free with proper treatment, yet many remain undiagnosed.

Epilepsy is significantly more prevalent in autistic individuals, with estimates ranging from 11% to 30%, especially among females and those with learning disabilities. Shared genetic factors, including conditions like Rett syndrome and Fragile X syndrome, may explain this connection.

Epilepsy is a spectrum condition, meaning the experience and frequency of seizures vary widely from person to person. Some may experience brief lapses in awareness, while others might have convulsions or loss of consciousness.

Equality Act 2010 ⚖️

The Equality Act 2010 is a crucial UK law that protects individuals from discrimination based on nine protected characteristics, including disability, which covers autism. It requires organisations – such as public bodies, employers, and service providers – to provide equal treatment and access for autistic individuals through measures like reasonable adjustments. These may include adapting communication methods or creating quiet spaces to address sensory needs.

The Act prohibits both direct and indirect discrimination. Direct discrimination occurs when someone is treated unfairly due to their autistic identity, such as being denied a job purely on that basis. Indirect discrimination arises when universal policies or practices disproportionately disadvantage autistic people, such as, for example, rigid communication protocols that fail to account for non-speaking communication styles.

Although the Act aims to protect, critics highlight challenges in its implementation and inconsistent enforcement. Neurodivergent individuals often face the burden of proving their need for adjustments. For instance, an autistic employee overwhelmed by bright lights or noise may request changes like dimmer lighting or a quieter workspace but is required to provide medical evidence and navigate lengthy processes with their management. This can be exhausting and expose them to scrutiny or disbelief. While the Act mandates reasonable adjustments, the gap between its theoretical protections and practical experiences can increase stress and feelings of exclusion.

Practical outcomes also vary widely, and awareness among employers and service providers is inconsistent. Critics advocate for stronger enforcement mechanisms and better training for organisations to ensure the Act's protections translate into meaningful change.

Eugenics 🚫

Eugenics is a controversial and harmful concept rooted in the belief that certain human traits, including neurological ones, are more desirable than others. This ideology promotes the notion that society should control human reproduction to 'improve' the population by encouraging reproduction among individuals with 'preferred' traits and discouraging or preventing it among those with traits deemed undesirable. Historically, eugenics has been associated with oppressive policies like forced sterilisation, marriage restrictions, and even genocide, particularly targeting disabled, neurodivergent, and marginalised people. Eugenics disregards the inherent value of human diversity, undermining the rights and dignity of individuals. For neurodivergent people, eugenics is especially damaging, as it reinforces the false idea that only certain types of minds are worthy of existence or respect.

European Union Disability Strategy 2021–2030 ⚖️

The EU Disability Strategy 2021–2030 is a key framework designed to promote the full inclusion and equal rights of disabled people across Europe. The strategy builds on previous efforts and emphasises accessibility, equality, and the empowerment of disabled individuals in all aspects of life. It aims to remove barriers to participation in society by focusing on areas such as employment, education, and social inclusion, ensuring that disabled people can lead independent lives. The strategy also aligns with the broader European commitment to human rights, particularly through the implementation of the United Nations Convention on the Rights of Persons With Disabilities (UNCRPD). Importantly, the strategy seeks to challenge societal prejudices and improve public attitudes towards disability, shifting focus towards equality and active participation rather than seeing disability as a deficit or a limitation.

European Union Employment Equality Directive (Council Directive 2000/78/EC) ⚖️

The EU Employment Equality Directive (Council Directive 2000/78/EC) is a European Union legal framework that establishes a comprehensive legal framework to promote equal treatment in employment and occupation across EU member states. It prohibits discrimination on various grounds, including disability, and mandates that all member states must take measures to ensure workplace equality. For autistic people and other neurodivergent individuals, this directive is essential because it requires employers to provide reasonable accommodations, enabling them to thrive in their roles without being disabled by the environment.

Excoriation disorder 🧠 🌿

Also known as 'dermatillomania' or 'skin picking disorder,' excoriation disorder involves repetitive, compulsive skin-picking that can cause sores, scarring, or infections. It is often linked to stress, anxiety, and sensory discomfort, serving as a coping mechanism for overwhelming feelings. However, it can create a cycle of guilt and frustration due to its difficulty to control and its visible, painful consequences. Individuals with this disorder pick their skin an average of 2–3 times per day, typically for 10–30 minutes.

Excoriation disorder is frequently misunderstood and stigmatised. It is wrongly seen as self-inflicted harm stemming from poor self-control rather than an unconscious response to mental health difficulties. Understanding and compassionate support, rather than judgement, are essential, as is addressing the root causes, such as stress, anxiety, and sensory overwhelm.

Executive functioning

Executive functioning refers to a set of cognitive processes that enable individuals to manage and organise tasks, regulate emotions, and adapt to changing environments, circumstances, and demands. These processes, which are influenced by anxiety and levels of physical and mental energy levels, include working memory, cognitive flexibility, and self-control. Autistic individuals often experience differences in executive functioning, impacting their ability to plan, manage time, and adapt to disruptions in routine. Such challenges can lead to increased anxiety, particularly in environments that demand rapid decision-making or frequent changes. For example, an autistic student might excel in completing assignments when given clear instructions and a structured schedule. However, if a teacher suddenly changes a deadline or introduces new expectations without warning, the student may experience significant stress and struggle to adjust, not because of a lack of ability, but due to the executive functioning demands of adapting to the unexpected change.

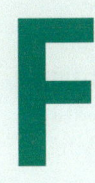

Fake cures ⃠

Fake cures describe unscientific and often harmful treatments falsely marketed as remedies for autism. These exploit the hope and desperation of vulnerable families, perpetuating the harmful notion that autism needs 'fixing.' Such 'treatments' include dangerous practices, unregulated supplements, and therapies claiming to 'reverse' autism without legitimate evidence. Social media platforms, especially Facebook and WhatsApp, amplify misinformation. A particularly alarming example is chlorine dioxide, marketed as 'Miracle Mineral Solution' (MMS) but effectively industrial bleach. The United States' FDA has issued multiple warnings about the risks of consuming MMS, yet its use persists in some communities, causing severe harm and, in some cases, death. These practices also serve to perpetuate the stigma of autism. The use of such practices should be universally outlawed, and instead of seeking cures, efforts should be directed towards understanding, acceptance, and providing meaningful support for autistic individuals to thrive.

Felt stigma 🌿 ⃠

Felt stigma refers to the internalisation of negative societal stereotypes, causing individuals to expect rejection or judgement based on their identity. Autistic people often experience this more intensely than neurotypicals, anticipating marginalisation or misunderstanding. This can lead to self-imposed limitations, anxiety, depression, reduced self esteem, and social withdrawal due to fear of prejudice. Anticipating stigma activates brain regions linked to social pain and rejection, indicating a neurobiological component to this distress. Felt stigma is especially damaging as it persists even without overt (enacted) stigma, rooted in past experiences or societal awareness. Peer-led support and stigma resistance initiatives play a crucial role in mitigating its harmful effects.

Fibromyalgia 💬

Fibromyalgia is a long-term neurological condition characterised by widespread pain and heightened sensitivity to touch. People with fibromyalgia often experience chronic fatigue, difficulty with memory or concentration (sometimes referred to as 'fibro fog'), and sleep disturbances. Symptoms can also include stiffness, headaches, and irritable bowel syndrome. The exact cause remains unclear although research shows altered brain connectivity in areas linked to pain processing and sensory integration, supporting the theory of central sensitisation — where the nervous system becomes hypersensitive to pain signals, amplifying sensations that would normally be mild or harmless.

Fibromyalgia is not associated with structural damage or inflammation in muscles and joints, making it difficult to diagnose through standard medical tests. Instead, diagnosis is typically based on a person's symptoms and a process of eliminating other potential causes of pain. However, recent studies using machine learning algorithms on functional MRI data have shown promising accuracy in distinguishing fibromyalgia patients from healthy individuals, offering hope for more reliable diagnostic tools.

Filicide 🚫

Filicide is the tragic act of a parent killing their own child. This issue disproportionately affects disabled children, including autistic children. Cases of filicide are sometimes wrongly framed in the media and public discourse in a way that shifts blame away from the perpetrator and instead places focus on the child's supposed burdens. This dangerous narrative contributes to further dehumanisation of disabled people by implying that their lives are less valuable or that the parent's actions were somehow understandable. Filicide is an outcome of societal failure — failing to provide necessary support and acceptance for individuals and their families. It reflects the ongoing issue of ableism and the harmful belief that disabled lives are less worth living and the importance of challenging ableist narratives in media, healthcare, and public policy.

Fragile X 💬

Fragile X is a genetic condition caused by a mutation in the FMR1 gene, affecting brain development and often associated with learning differences and neurodivergence. It occurs across all populations, with a global prevalence estimated between 0.01% and 0.018%. While often linked to intellectual disabilities and developmental differences, understanding Fragile X through the neurodiversity paradigm highlights it as a variation in cognitive functioning rather than a deficit.

People with Fragile X may experience heightened sensory sensitivity, social communication challenges, and, in some cases, strengths in pattern recognition, visual-spatial tasks, and attention to detail. These abilities deserve recognition, and with acceptance, understanding, and tailored support, individuals with Fragile X can lead enriched and fulfilling lives.

Functional neurological disorder 💬

Functional neurological disorder (FND) refers to a condition where individuals experience neurological presentations such as motor or sensory issues (e.g., limb weakness, tremors, seizures) that are not easily explained by typical medical tests or structural brain damage. It is often misunderstood as purely psychological, but recent insights show it involves a complex interaction between the brain's functioning and psychological factors. While the presentation of FND can appear similar to those of other neurological types, FND exists on its own as a valid diagnosis, and its challenges are genuine and distressing. Specialised physiotherapy and psychological therapy can be effective in increasing the quality of life among those experiencing FND.

Functioning labels 🚫

Functioning labels refer to the problematic categorisation of autistic people based on perceived abilities, often described as 'high-functioning' or 'low-functioning.' These labels oversimplify the complex and dynamic nature of support needs, leading to harmful misunderstandings. 'High-functioning' is often used to dismiss the struggles faced by autistic people who may appear more independent, while 'low-functioning' reinforces the misconception that individuals with more visible support needs lack capabilities. Both labels fail to account for the fluctuating nature of autistic experiences and do not reflect the individual's true needs. This binary view perpetuates stigma and dehumanisation, reducing an individual's worth to their ability to function within a neurotypical framework rather than acknowledging their unique ways of interacting with the world. Ultimately, autistic people may experience varying levels of support across different situations, and functioning labels undermine the principle of neurodivergent acceptance.

Further education colleges 🏢

Further education colleges in the United Kingdom provide a vital pathway for those who wish to continue their education beyond the age of 16, offering a broad range of qualifications and training opportunities, serving students with varying needs, whether they are pursuing academic studies, vocational training, or skill development for employment. These institutions also exist in other countries under different names: in the United States, they are referred to as 'community colleges'; in Australia, they are known as 'technical and further education' institutions; in France, they are called 'lycées professionnels'; in Germany, they are referred to as 'berufsschulen'; and in India, they are often called 'industrial training institutes.' Many further education colleges are inclusive, aiming to support neurodivergent students, including autistic people, by offering tailored resources and environments that support different learning styles and sensory needs.

G

Global developmental delay

Global developmental delay is a term used to describe children under the age of five who exhibit significant delays – measured against the expected milestones of typically developing children – across multiple developmental domains, including cognitive, motor, language, and social skills. Unlike specific developmental differences, global developmental delay serves as an initial umbrella diagnosis, signalling the need for further evaluation to identify an underlying or more specific diagnosis or diagnoses.

This broad classification can facilitate early support but may also obscure specific needs and strengths of the individual. The word 'delay' itself can risk focusing attention on perceived shortcomings rather than celebrating the individuality and strengths of each child. These delays are not necessarily indicative of a deficit but often reflect differences in the pace and nature of development.

Gustatory sense

The gustatory system is responsible for the perception of taste, primarily through taste buds on the tongue. Autistic individuals often experience taste differently from non-autistic people. Some may be hypersensitive, finding certain tastes overwhelmingly intense, while others may be hyposensitive, requiring stronger or more varied flavours to detect taste. These sensory differences often influence food preferences and dietary habits, leading to selective eating.

Despite this, people with gustatory sensitivities are frequently labelled 'fussy eaters,' a term that dismisses the genuine sensory experiences shaping their eating habits. For those with heightened or reduced taste sensitivity, certain flavours or textures can be overpowering or barely noticeable. These responses are not about choice or stubbornness but reflect natural variations in sensory processing. Mislabelling them as 'fussy' can cause anxiety around food and undermine their needs. Greater understanding and acceptance of these differences are essential for providing meaningful support rather than judgement.

H

Hand flapping

Hand flapping is a form of stimming (self-stimulatory behaviour) used to regulate sensory input, express emotions, or manage overwhelming situations. It typically involves rapid hand or finger movements, varying in frequency and intensity.

This behaviour serves important functions, including self-regulation, emotional management, comfort, focus, and grounding, particularly during sensory overload or anxiety. In neurodivergent-affirming spaces, hand flapping is recognised as a natural part of human variation, not something to be suppressed or viewed negatively.

Hate crime 🚫

A hate crime is a criminal act motivated by prejudice against characteristics such as race, ethnicity, sexuality, religion, disability, or neurological identity. For neurodivergent people, these crimes often stem from stereotypes and stigma surrounding their identity. Such crimes can be direct or indirect. Direct hate crimes involve explicit acts of aggression, such as verbal abuse, physical assault, or harassment specifically targeting an individual because of their neurodivergent identity. Indirect hate crimes may include discriminatory policies, exclusionary practices, or environments designed in ways that marginalise neurodivergent people, such as failing to make reasonable workplace adjustments or enforcing rules that disproportionately disadvantage them.

Hate crimes cause significant harm – not just to individuals but to entire communities – by propagating fear, deepening social exclusion, and causing emotional and psychological damage. For neurodivergent people who also belong to other marginalised groups, they often face multiple layers of discrimination, making them particularly vulnerable to hate crimes.

Head banging

Head banging is a sensory-seeking behaviour that can occur when individuals experience sensory overload, unmet needs, or overwhelming emotions. It can serve as a form of self-regulation, helping individuals manage intense feelings or communicate distress when other communication methods are unavailable. For autistic people, who may experience heightened or dulled sensory input, head banging can provide physical sensations or reduce sensory chaos. It is more commonly observed in autistic individuals with co-occurring intellectual disabilities.

Rather than being a 'challenging behaviour,' head-banging is a 'behaviour that challenges' due to unmet needs and heightened stress. Support involves identifying and addressing underlying causes such as sensory overwhelm, anxiety, or pain, while creating a safe and understanding environment. Minimising sensory triggers and offering alternative self-soothing and communication methods can help reduce the reliance on head banging as a coping mechanism.

High-pressure socialising

High-pressure socialising refers to social situations where the expectation to engage and conform to certain social norms is intense. These situations can be particularly challenging for autistic people, who may process social interactions differently from neurotypical individuals. In such environments, there can be strong unspoken expectations around speed of response, non-speaking cues, or particular conversational styles, which do not account for neurodivergent communication styles. The pressure to fit into these rigid social frameworks often leads to masking, exhaustion, anxiety, and sensory overload for many autistics.

Homeschooling

Homeschooling involves educating a child outside conventional school systems, often tailored to meet their unique learning and sensory needs. This approach can be particularly valuable for neurodivergent children who may find traditional classroom settings overwhelming or unaccommodating. The flexibility of homeschooling allows for a learning environment adapted to a child's sensory and emotional needs, with regular breaks, sensory-friendly spaces, and a personalised curriculum. It empowers families to prioritise learning in ways that align with a child's strengths and interests. Despite its name, homeschooling still includes opportunities for social interaction and community engagement in a safe and inclusive way, making the word 'home' somewhat misleading.

However, homeschooling is often stigmatised, with misconceptions about isolation or poor parenting. It also demands significant time, resources, and dedication from caregivers, making it impractical for some families. Support from authorities and organisations remains essential to ensure homeschooling families are not marginalised or overlooked simply because their children are educated outside traditional systems.

Human Rights Act 1998 ⚖️

The Human Rights Act 1998 is a cornerstone of UK law, incorporating the European Convention on Human Rights into domestic legislation. It safeguards against discrimination and advances equality, benefiting autistic and other neurodivergent individuals. Key provisions like the right to respect for private and family life (Article 8) and protection from discrimination (Article 14) support advocacy for equal treatment and accessibility in healthcare, education, and social services.

Despite its promise, these rights are not always consistently upheld. Marginalised groups, including neurodivergent people, often face complex legal challenges to enforce their rights. The Act's effectiveness relies on public awareness and institutional accountability, which can vary widely, limiting its impact in daily life.

For example, the right to education without discrimination (Article 14 with Article 2 of Protocol No. 1) may be breached if an autistic student is denied reasonable adjustments in a mainstream school. This could lead to exclusion or placement in an unsuitable educational setting. Challenging such failures frequently involves navigating intricate legal systems, exposing gaps in the Act's implementation and leaving autistic individuals at a disadvantage in asserting their rights to equitable access and support.

Humiliation 🚫

Humiliation is an intense emotional experience where an individual's dignity or status is forcibly reduced, often through actions intended to degrade them in front of others. Unlike private shame or embarrassment, humiliation typically involves public exposure, with an audience witnessing the act. It differs from trauma by centring on the intentional stripping of dignity, often used as a form of control or punishment.

For neurodivergent individuals, humiliation can have a particularly profound impact. Differences in social communication, sensory processing, and emotional regulation often make them more vulnerable to being misunderstood or unfairly targeted. Autistic people, for example, might not respond in socially expected ways during humiliating situations – they may struggle to make eye contact, remain silent, or react in ways others misinterpret as indifference, defiance, or overreaction. These differences can unintentionally escalate the situation or lead to further mistreatment, amplifying their distress.

A history of marginalisation and repeated exposure to humiliating experiences – whether in school, the workplace, or social settings – can result in deep-seated anxiety, depression, and social withdrawal. These effects are often compounded by societal attitudes that pathologise or dismiss neurodivergent identities.

Understanding and addressing the unique ways neurodivergent individuals experience and process humiliation are essential for creating spaces where dignity is protected and emotional well-being is prioritised.

Hybrid learning

Hybrid learning blends in-person and online education, offering flexibility for neurodivergent students, including autistic individuals, to access environments suited to their needs. It accommodates diverse learning styles by providing multiple ways to engage with content – visual, auditory, or written – supporting those who prefer alternative modes of communication or sensory input.

This approach emphasises personal agency, reducing the pressures of traditional classroom settings and allowing autistic students to better manage sensory overwhelm and focus more effectively. By adapting to individual support needs, hybrid learning promotes inclusivity over a one-size-fits-all model.

Hyperacusis

Hyperacusis is an increased sensitivity to everyday sounds, where noises others find tolerable can feel overwhelming or painful. Autistic people are more likely to experience this due to sensory processing differences, making busy or noisy environments particularly challenging. Hyperacusis is a neurological response, not a preference, and managing it often involves noise-cancelling headphones, quiet spaces, or other accommodations to reduce sensory overload. It is distinct from tinnitus, which involves perceiving internal sounds like ringing or buzzing that are not externally present. While hyperacusis relates to external noise sensitivity, tinnitus concerns phantom sounds disrupting auditory perception.

Hypercontrol

The term hypercontrol refers to the conscious or sub-conscious need some autistic individuals may feel to manage or dominate various aspects of their environment and personal routines in an effort to reduce anxiety and self-regulate. This tendency can manifest as strict adherence to schedules, particular routines, or an overwhelming focus on maintaining order and predictability. Hypercontrol often arises from an autistic person's desire to mitigate the overwhelming sensory input and unpredictability they might face in a neurotypical world. It is not a negative trait to be 'corrected' but rather a coping mechanism for managing an often hostile or overstimulating environment. Overemphasis on forcing flexibility in these areas can cause emotional distress, underscoring the importance of understanding, respect, and creating supportive spaces where neurodivergent people can feel safe without needing to rely on hypercontrol.

Hyperempathy 💬 🌿

Hyperempathy is an intense sensitivity to others' emotions, where individuals deeply feel and sometimes absorb these emotions as their own. Despite the outdated belief that autistic people lack empathy, hyperempathy is common among autistic individuals. This heightened emotional resonance can be overwhelming and make it difficult to separate their own feelings from those of others. Despite its significance, hyperempathy remains under-recognised in standard autism diagnostic criteria.

However, hyperempathy does not always equate to emotional literacy – the ability to identify, understand, or articulate emotions. Many autistic people experience alexithymia, which can complicate recognising or labelling feelings, even when emotions are intensely felt. Hyperempathy refers to the depth and intensity of emotional experience, not necessarily the ability to make sense of it.

This sensitivity can result in being profoundly affected by others' distress, sometimes to the point of emotional overwhelm, disrupting daily activities or responsibilities. While it can lead to deeply meaningful connections, it may also impede interactions if the person struggles to process the emotions they're absorbing. Additionally, it can increase susceptibility to emotional manipulation, especially by narcissistic individuals.

IN MY OWN WORDS: BEN BREAUX

I am a hyperempathic autistic. Sometimes this intensely emotional experience can lead to a physical response in my body, which can even cause me immense discomfort. They feel like emotional waves that are hard to distinguish from my own emotions sometimes. It can be overwhelming not knowing if I'm upset or someone else is. I don't often feel the emotions of strangers but family and close friends can really impact me. Namely my mom, as we are so close. Our emotions are so intertwined. I can feel her joy from miles away, which can make her absence difficult to manage. Recently my sister had a big accomplishment that my family was so excited about – possibly no one more so than my mom. Her excitement and joy over this stayed with me for days. It is a very treasured feeling.

When the emotions are negative, this can be incredibly difficult to navigate. It feels like a sudden jolt of emotion, as if it's been transmitted to me rather than coming from within. It can be difficult to explain what this feels like because it feels like any emotion I might feel but very clearly not my own. I am simultaneously experiencing it and observing it. The negative emotions

are harder to distinguish from my own and far more uncomfortable. If I feel a negative emotion from someone long enough or if it's strong enough, it begins to become my own emotion. I will feel anxious or stressed or angry but with no internal cause. What I find most difficult about these moments is that because the emotion didn't come from me, it is harder to help myself feel better. It is easier to help the person struggling with the emotion – find a way to make them feel better – because once their emotion is calmed, I can calm myself. Distance is occasionally helpful but not always possible.

On the whole, I consider being hyperempathic to definitely be a more positive attribute. I like being able to form such strong attachments with the people in my life. The positives far outweigh the negatives. I find that with my co-regulation partners, the part that hurts me the most is when they leave. I form such strong bonds with them that when they leave, it can feel like I've lost a part of myself. We are so connected and that enriches my life in so many ways. I can only really see the positives in my hyperempathy. It makes all of the relationships in my life so much stronger, and I wouldn't give that up for anything. It can be difficult to manage so many feelings alongside my own, but it is so worth it. To be this connected to the people in my life is a gift.

Hyperfocus

Hyperfocus is a state of intense, deep concentration on a specific task or interest, often experienced by neurodivergent individuals, especially autistic and AuDHD people. Unlike general focus, hyperfocus often involves becoming so absorbed that time, external stimuli, and other responsibilities fade into the background. This can result in exceptional productivity, expertise, and fulfilment when aligned with personal passions but may also cause challenges when switching tasks or maintaining self-care routines.

Rather than being a flaw, hyperfocus reflects monotropism – a tendency to focus deeply on singular interests. It can bring joy, achievement, and a profound sense of purpose but may disrupt essential activities like eating or sleeping if left unchecked. Supporting hyperfocus involves minimising interruptions, recognising its value, and creating environments that allow it to flourish. For example, teachers can allow students to delve deeply into their dedicated interests during learning activities, and employers can provide quiet workspaces to minimise distractions.

IN MY OWN WORDS: ANDREW KINGSLOW

Hyperfocus for me is a way to shut out the cacophony that soundtracks my life. I have to admit that much of this noise is internalised as negative thoughts that try to knock me off my daily routine. As an autistic person with strong ADHD traits, I tread a fine balance between order and disorder. During an ADHD cycle, the autistic part of me struggles with the disarray and mess. Conversely, during an autistic cycle, I can't tolerate environments that are visually and audibly loud.

There is, however, a slight centre of this Venn diagram where both versions of me find peace, and that is in a state of hyperfocus. I'd go so far as to say it's a form of stimming because it helps me regulate. For example, in my early music career, I took up the piano and, within a year, reached grade 8 standard, gaining a scholarship to a prestigious music school. Another example would be spending eight hours entering code into a computer for little to no return other than the satisfaction of completing the task. I was obsessed with 0–60 times of cars and would remember the decimal points, along with various other stats. Looking back, there was comfort in having this knowledge in my mind. Sometimes, I'd repeat those figures in my head like a mantra – perhaps another way to regulate.

In later life, I chose a vocation as a music producer that enables me to be in the room and not in the room at the same time. Let me explain: I operate as a technician and programmer, allowing me to focus on computer-based tasks whenever I don't have the energy to interact with people – sometimes to the point where I miss meals and bathroom breaks for hours on end!

On the downside, it is incredibly difficult to deal with not being able to carry out my special interests, which tend to be the subjects of my hyperfocus. The challenge of having that taken away is massive and can be almost meltdown-inducing. The sense of loss and frustration when I am unable to engage in these interests is overwhelming.

Ultimately, hyperfocus allows me to quiet my mind and tunnel in on something that provides an escape, a relief from anxiety, and a sense of worth.

Hyperlexia

Hyperlexia is an intense, early fascination with reading, often seen in neurodivergent individuals, particularly autistic people. Unlike typically developing children, hyperlexic individuals can decode written words exceptionally early, sometimes even as toddlers. However, this skill often accompanies difficulties in understanding spoken language, social communication, or reading comprehension, meaning they may not necessarily grasp the meanings behind the words. While hyperlexia can be a powerful strength, supporting language comprehension and communication is essential. It is also sometimes linked with an advanced ability to understand numbers, known as 'hypernumeracy,' and it may suggest a broader strength in pattern recognition and symbolic reasoning among autistic people. This profile can lead to exceptional abilities in areas such as mathematics and data analysis.

IN MY OWN WORDS: LYRIC RIVERA

I am hyperlexic. Hyperlexic People are a unique group. We often display exceptional early reading skills, surpassing the expected skill level for our age and grade.

At different times in my life, being hyperlexic has been both a blessing and a curse, but primarily (for me), my hyperlexic mind has been a gift.

My spoken comprehension and abilities have always been far lower than my reading and writing abilities, which tested "off the charts" in elementary school. (The gap between the two is much smaller and less noticeable now than when I was a kid.)

Many of us embark on our reading journey at a remarkably young age. This early proficiency is often accompanied by an insatiable hunger for reading, devouring books and exploring language in all its diverse forms.

Reading was my very first Autistic Focused Interest (or Special Interest).

I taught myself to read at the age of one and a half, surprising the adults in my life by one day reading out names on a map from the back seat of the car while we were on a road trip.

Nobody realized that the infant in the back seat had taken it upon themselves to study, and the adults were surprised and amused to learn that I'd somehow acquired this ability at such a young age.

While it's a fascinating trait, being hyperlexic can also pose significant challenges in our lives, often leading to misunderstandings or overlooked struggles.

For example, in school, though I was a proficient reader (testing off the charts in my reading level), I was anxious and unable to read out loud in front of my peers, experiencing selective mutism from the anxiety and pressure of reading with an audience.

Because I could read (well) on my own, my struggle reading in front of others was seen as a "refusal" (needing punishment) instead of an "inability" (requiring support), like it really was.

Many teachers felt that because I could read to myself VERY WELL, I should be able to master reading out loud and do other tasks, as well as every school subject, with the same ease.

I was never a "well-rounded" student.

Regardless, being gifted in one academic area meant teachers expected more from me in every area (even if I didn't have more to give) and had less patience for my struggles whenever I had them.

Sometimes, it feels as if the person who does my writing and the person who does my speaking are two completely different people.

Because my spoken comprehension and the way I speak are not at the same level as my reading and writing skills (and this was even more noticeable when I was younger), in school, teachers frequently accused me of "cheating" when I turned in essays and book reports because I "don't talk like" my papers are written.

Beyond reading, hyperlexics tend to have a unique relationship with language.

We might obsess over word origins, etymology, grammar, and syntax.

We often notice patterns and connections between words that others might miss.

This linguistic curiosity has led me down rabbit holes of exploration, from deciphering ancient scripts to creating my own languages in middle school.

My hyperlexia allows me to excel in written storytelling. I use my linguistic agility to connect with others and convey complex ideas through text (or scripts I read in video format).

My love for words, language, and books has enabled me to become a best-selling author and contributor to multiple books related to Autism and NeuroDiversity.

On the one hand, our love for language grants us access to a rich inner world of imagination, creativity, and expression. However, hyperlexia can also be overwhelming and isolating.

Our intense focus on language can lead to social difficulties as we struggle to disengage from the words and text around us, or it can cause us to be misinterpreted by the people around us.

We may constantly transcribe the world, decode every conversation, and analyze every written word. This constant mental activity can be exhausting.

But even with the pain and misunderstandings, I wouldn't trade this experience of being hyperlexic for anything.

Hyperosmia

Hyperosmia refers to an acute or heightened sense of smell, meaning that individuals experience odours more intensely than the general population. It can lead to discomfort or even distress when exposed to strong or unpleasant odours that others might not notice or find tolerable. This heightened olfactory sensitivity can be a common experience among neurodivergent people, including autistic individuals given their varying sensory profiles, and hyperosmia can be one aspect of this.

Hyperphantasia

Hyperphantasia is the exceptionally vivid ability to visualise images, concepts, or scenarios in one's mind. Rather than simply being a passive experience, hyperphantasia can involve rich, detailed, and lifelike imaginings that can influence creativity, memory, and problem-solving. It stands in contrast to aphantasia, in which mental imagery is absent or significantly reduced. While hyperphantasia may be highly enriching, providing intense inner experiences, it can also be overwhelming in certain contexts, such as when the vividness of mental images or scenarios becomes intrusive. The experience and impact of hyperphantasia will vary widely, making it a point of curiosity and research within neurodivergent communities.

Hyperplasticity

Hyperplasticity describes to the brain's increased ability to change, adapt, and form new connections throughout life (the process of 'neuroplasticity'). In neurodivergent contexts, particularly within the autistic community, hyperplasticity can be understood as a more flexible and heightened neural adaptability. This allows for heightened sensitivity to new experiences and environments. While this can support creative problem-solving, effective memory, and unique thought processes, it can also make autistic people more vulnerable to sensory overload and stress. Understanding hyperplasticity helps illustrate that autistic neurology represents a natural variation in how human brains can adapt and engage with the world.

Hypersensitivity and hyposensitivity

Hypersensitivity and hyposensitivity describe how some neurodivergent people, including autistic individuals, process sensory input differently. Hypersensitivity involves heightened sensitivity, where stimuli like sounds, lights, or textures can feel overwhelming or distressing. In contrast, hyposensitivity refers to reduced sensitivity, leading individuals to seek stronger stimuli, such as deep pressure or particular sound patterns, for comfort or engagement. A person can experience both simultaneously across different senses – for example, being hypersensitive to loud sounds while hyposensitive to touch. These sensory experiences can also fluctuate throughout the day or in different environments, adding complexity to how autistic individuals interact with the world.

Identification vs diagnosis 🧠 💧

The distinction between identification and diagnosis highlights two different ways individuals come to understand their autistic identity. Identification refers to recognising and accepting one's autistic identity, often through self-reflection or community validation. This process can bring personal relief and empowerment as individuals come to understand their neurology in a self-affirming way. However, it may be unfairly viewed as less valid by others, especially services, leading to stigma or dismissal of lived experiences.

Diagnosis, on the other hand, involves a formal medical assessment that labels characteristics through a clinical lens. While it can provide access to support, the medical framing of autism as a 'disorder,' and the diagnostic tools used, which often pathologise autism, can reinforce stigma.

Many individuals prefer identification for its self-affirming approach, while others pursue diagnosis for practical benefits and external validation. For some, identification leads to seeking a formal diagnosis, while, for others, diagnosis prompts deeper self-acceptance. Both paths are equally valid, reflecting diverse ways people affirm their autistic identity.

IN MY OWN WORDS: KOSJENKA PETEK

It's complicated. I'd rather not delve into it. Why? Because the vast and often highly antagonistic divide between professionals, the autistic community, and parents is distressing to me. Yet, as someone who is autistic, I find it all feels oddly straightforward. We understand the diagnostic criteria. I fully grasp the importance of differential diagnosis, especially for those of us who've experienced early trauma or have overlapping mental health conditions. But the discourse surrounding the merging of ex-Asperger's syndrome with autism spectrum condition feels militant, aggressive, and, at times, incomprehensible.

DOI: 10.4324/9781003477297-9

I was the third adult woman in Croatia to be diagnosed with autism. This was in 2018. Rumour has it the first woman diagnosed, under what was then called Asperger's syndrome, received her diagnosis during the Yugoslavian era. The second woman, Zrinka, had to travel to Italy for her assessment because Croatia didn't have adult diagnostic teams or trained professionals at the time. In fact, undiagnosed autistic adults in Croatia were almost invisible, existing only on Twitter or in obscure Facebook groups like Autism Inclusivity.

In 2018, I too went to Italy for a diagnosis. It was after my third experience of being bullied at work, the breakdown of my second marriage, a history of grooming and sexual exploitation, and two decades spent in a cult – all while raising a diagnosed autistic child. I didn't know what was wrong with me, only that *something* was. Three instances of workplace bullying, and I was the common denominator? It had to be me. I thought, *I must make people want to do something to me.*

To support my autistic child, I read every book I could find. In those books, I saw myself. But admitting I might be autistic? That was much harder. I wrote countless emails to autism parent NGOs in Croatia, asking for help, advice, or even just a kind word. No one responded. Not once in five years. Occasionally, I revisit those old emails to see how I sounded. *Couldn't they hear a woman in pain? A human being in need of help?*

The day I received my diagnosis felt like my second birthday. It was a rebirth. My diagnostician was wonderful – knowledgeable, tactful, and compassionate. Though he wasn't a woman and didn't have experiential knowledge of what it's like to be one, he had cognitive empathy and a deep understanding of autism in women. He explained *me* to *myself*: why I feel like I don't belong, why I've always imagined an alien mothership might come for me, why I've experienced unwanted advances, why I have meltdowns. He showed me that I was normal. Autistic-normal.

But the diagnosis wasn't without its consequences. The day after receiving it, I realised that, in some ways, nothing had changed. My life would remain the same: always on guard, always hiding, shielding, protecting myself. *"Same as it ever was,"* as David Byrne sings. I had a profound emotional breakdown in Rome and attempted to end my life by jumping off a bridge. My child and my friend were there and witnessed it. That moment is now a reality we all live with, something we will carry for the rest of our lives.

Did I self-diagnose before my official diagnosis? No. I'm from Croatia, where disability justice, self-organisation, and awareness of self-diagnosis lag 15 to 20 years behind much of the world. It wasn't part of my cultural belief system. I needed validation from a professional. Over time, I've learned to forgive myself for that need.

It's not just autism. I also struggle to recognise sensations in my body, which has led to multiple ER visits and even emergency surgeries because I didn't realise my symptoms were serious. So, yes, I understand why I needed an official diagnosis.

However, even an official diagnosis from a renowned autism centre in Italy means little where I live. My physician doesn't consider me autistic. Autism professionals in Croatia doubt my diagnosis – despite having never met or spoken to me. They've only seen me on TV. I practiced delivering my lines eloquently and with humour for a television interview, following the advice of the interviewer. But I wasn't "autistic enough" on screen. And because I'm a woman, this perception was even more pronounced.

The backlash was severe. I've been bullied, abused, and even threatened online for appearing in the media as an officially diagnosed autistic woman. One man fixated on me, orchestrating cascades of online abuse, with autism parent NGOs joining in. The fear from his threats drove me to psychotherapy and made me dread both going to work and returning home late at night.

As I type this in October 2024, Croatia still doesn't have an official protocol for diagnosing autistic adults. One is in the works, but the process is slow. Even among the handful of professionals who identify and diagnose autistic adults – who use tools like the ADOS test and make differential diagnoses – their work is often dismissed by their peers. The semi-official stance is that autism in Croatian adults, particularly women, is "overdiagnosed."

Given all this, whether someone self-diagnoses or receives an official diagnosis from a registered professional hardly matters in Croatia, does it?

Still, there is a community here. We've organised ourselves. We host soirees, therapy groups, autism picnics, movie nights, conferences, and even partner with the Croatian Union of Associations for Autism. They listen to us, help us build advocacy skills, and amplify our message. Together, we're building bridges – on our terms. That autonomy and freedom make me proud.

One last thing for readers outside Eastern Europe: Croatia hasn't implemented ICD-11 yet. Our medical staff still rely on DSM-IV and ICD–10. So if you meet a Croatian who says they have Asperger's, please be kind. Autism spectrum disorder hasn't fully arrived here, and autistic women like me still remain, in many ways, vague and mythological creatures.

Identity-first language

Identity-first language prioritises an individual's identifying characteristic, such as 'autistic person' instead of 'person with autism.' This reflects the view that neurodivergence is an intrinsic part of identity, integral to who they are rather than a separate or secondary attribute. This approach is typically used with other core identities; for example, someone might say they are a 'Chinese person' rather than 'a person with Chinese ethnicity.'

Person-first language, by contrast, aligns with a medical model, often used for temporary or negative conditions. For instance, we say 'he has cancer' because it is negative, treatable, and potentially curable. Neurodivergence, however, belongs to identity categories, akin to ethnicity, gender, or nationality, rather than medical conditions.

IN MY OWN WORDS: BEN BREAUX

I do NOT 'suffer from' autism – I am autistic, it is part of who I am. My autism does NOT need to be 'fixed.' My autism affects every part of my life. It is not my whole identity, but it does affect how I interact with people and the world around me. So, it is important to present it first in introductions. Also, it is an adjective that describes me and my behaviors. Autism is not a disease, and person-first language is what you use for something someone is trying to get rid of or beat, like COVID or an infection (person with COVID). No one cures their autism, and it's not something we can 'beat' or eliminate.' nor would I want to.

Illegal so-called 'cures' 🚫

This refers to treatments or remedies that falsely claim to cure autism, a neurological identity, which is neither an illness nor condition to be cured. These unscientific remedies, such as chlorine dioxide bleach, are not only ineffective but also extremely dangerous, causing severe health risks, including seizures, vomiting, and even death.

Beyond physical harm, these treatments cause lasting psychological trauma. Survivors often internalise damaging beliefs that they are fundamentally flawed or unacceptable, increasing risks of anxiety, internalised ableism, and suicidal ideation.

Advocates have long campaigned for these harmful practices to be universally illegal, mirroring existing legislation against fraudulent cancer treatments.

IN MY OWN WORDS: KOSJENKA PETEK

I've never quite understood why so many parents fall into the trap of trying to 'cure' autism.

Perhaps it's because autism is an invisible disability, leading us to believe it can somehow be eradicated, leaving behind a child 'without autism.' To this day, I'm not entirely sure. Even though I've volunteered at an autistic-led NGO and participated in countless online parent groups, I remain baffled by the number of parents who endlessly search for cures. It's devastating.

Looking back, I realise I became immersed in the cure narrative very early on.

In hindsight, I think it starts even before a child is born. The fear of autism is instilled first.

When I was a young woman planning my family, while at one of the best fertility clinics, I came across posts on prominent parenting forums. The message was clear: *"Don't vaccinate your child, or they will develop autism. Autism leaves you with a shell of a child, with nothing inside."*

Then there were the April Autism Day news reports from autism NGOs warning about the so-called 'French Scenario' – dire tales of parents struggling with autistic children in France. Those stories heightened my fears. Ultimately, they led me to make the decision not to vaccinate my child. Looking back, I ask myself, *how could I have been so naive?*

But I understand why. As a hopeful mother-to-be, desperate for the clinic's help after so many failed attempts to conceive, I was consumed by the desire to protect my child at all costs. My vulnerability was exploited.

When my child started showing signs of developing differently from his peers, autism never crossed our minds. After all, he hadn't been vaccinated, remember? So when we finally received his diagnosis – autism spectrum condition – it was a shock. We felt an overwhelming sense of self-blame.

Around that time, a health practitioner told us, *"You can do a lot. It depends on how well off you are."*

But what was this 'a lot' they mentioned? No one even gave us a pamphlet. No one directed us towards autism NGOs.

Instead, we turned to parent forums, where the chatter was relentless: *"Heavy metals aren't just in vaccines; they're everywhere. Start with a strict gluten- and lactose-free diet, bioresonance testing, and supplements. Then add MMS cleanses, iodine, and chelation."*

We followed their advice, and I still deeply regret it. We drastically restricted our child's diet. We put him — and ourselves — into impossible situations. We pushed beyond every healthy emotional, physical, and financial limit.

In those forums, being radical, strict, and unyielding was equated with being a responsible and caring parent: *"Don't let your child manipulate you into giving up! You have the power to save him."*

Every small shift — whether in sensory sensitivities, stimming, or routines — was treated as a victory just out of reach, as long as we stayed stricter and enforced more rules.

It caused us all immense grief and pain. Our family argued, blamed each other, and accused one another of failing our child. Relationships suffered across the board.

And why? Because people exploited our ignorance and vulnerability to sell their so-called cures for autism.

The turning point came before we considered trying MMS or chelation.
A loving friend in the USA sent me a copy of *NeuroTribes* by Steve Silberman. That book, and one mother's story within it, saved us. Shannon Des Roches Rosa wrote about her journey with her son Leo — a journey that echoed ours.

Through Shannon's story, I learned that the so-called cures and protocols dominating Balkan parent forums in 2016 and 2017 had already been debunked — some of them decades earlier! Her words helped me realise the harm we were causing. Shannon and her son Leo saved my son, Al.

Through *NeuroTribes*, I connected with Steve Silberman and Shannon on Twitter. From there, I discovered the wider autistic community — a diverse, opinionated, and loving group of people living the reality of autism every day.

I started listening.

And from them, I began to truly learn.

Imposter syndrome

Imposter syndrome is a psychological pattern where individuals doubt their accomplishments and fear being exposed as frauds, despite evidence of success or competence. It stems from an internalised belief of not belonging or being undeserving of achievements rather than actual ability. Neurodivergent people, particularly autistics, may experience this more intensely due to internalised societal stigma and neurotypical definitions of success. External pressures, such as group expectations and ableist attitudes, can amplify these feelings. Imposter syndrome is associated with increased stress, burnout, and reduced job satisfaction over time. Addressing it involves reframing self-worth, embracing neurodivergence, and creating environments that value diverse cognitive and social strengths.

Inclusive design

Inclusive design, sometimes referred to as universal design, creates environments, products, and systems that are accessible and usable by as many people as possible, regardless of age, ability, neurological identity, or circumstances. Rather than adding accessibility features as an afterthought, inclusivity is integrated from the start, ensuring that diverse needs are considered as a core principle rather than an optional extra.

This approach rejects the outdated divide between 'standard' and 'accessible' design, embedding equity and dignity into every stage of the design process. It actively challenges exclusionary practices by incorporating varied user perspectives and addressing sensory, cognitive, and physical differences.

Examples of inclusive design include modular lighting systems for personalised adjustments, acoustic features to reduce overwhelming background noise, and clear navigation systems with consistent visual cues, colour coding, and symbols for easier orientation. These elements not only address specific needs but also enhance usability for everyone.

Closely aligned with the social model of disability, inclusive design sees exclusion as a failure of environments and systems to accommodate diversity, not a reflection of individual 'limitations.' At its core, inclusive design does not just accommodate difference – it actively values it, creating spaces and systems where everyone can participate fully and authentically.

Inclusive education

Inclusive education embraces the principle that all students, including autistic and otherwise neurodivergent individuals, should learn together in the same age-appropriate classrooms and learning environments. Achieving this requires a cultural shift towards relationship-focused teaching, sensory-friendly spaces, and trauma-informed, co-regulation-based practices. Co-regulation strategies involve supportive processes by which one person helps another to manage their emotional and physiological state. This can include teachers and peers actively engaging in calming techniques, providing reassurance, and shaping an emotionally safe environment that ultimately creates a sense of security and trust.

Without inclusivity, autistic students often face bullying, exclusion, and heightened stress, while non-autistic peers miss opportunities to understand diverse ways of thinking. Collaboration with neurodivergent individuals in designing policies is essential for creating environments that prioritise acceptance, belonging, and holistic well-being for all students.

IN MY OWN WORDS: IQRA BABAR

There is a considerable amount to be mentioned regarding the state of education and its idea and praxis of inclusion. As it stands, inclusive education in the UK utilises terms such as SEN or SEND to single out disabled and neurodivergent pupils disguised as a means of provision and support. There is little acknowledgement, let alone the use of the term 'neurodiversity' or 'neurodivergent' in school policies or general schools, due to the overwhelming reliance on the pathology paradigm and the DSM as a means of measuring disability and neurodivergence.

The UK education system has fundamental issues, especially with how it supports disabled and neurodivergent students. As a primary school teacher, I've experienced these issues firsthand. Despite my love for education and learning, I find it difficult to feel fulfilled due to the overwhelming workload, high expectations, and rigid rules and policies. The term 'SEND,' for instance, used to refer to neurodivergent and disabled students, feels extremely inadequate and uncomfortable to me. This is due to the condescending nature behind the use of it. More often than not, it is used as a euphemism to, essentially, mock the child or view them as naughty, 'less than,' or academically flawed. It seems like the system struggles to simply acknowledge neurodiversity and disability without using negatively connoted language. This, in turn, makes practising teaching in mainstream schools difficult. For me, it has been a very tough start to my career knowing this, as well as simply being an auDHD worker. I constantly feel overwhelmed and struggle to keep up with the job's demands. Organization becomes difficult and the constant pressures from the job itself and those in power can make it feel suffocating. That's not to say that I don't love my field, I do, I adore working in education and being in this field, but, being on the 'front line' of it in the classroom is, at the very least, tough.

Additionally, the lack of mandatory training in understanding neurodiversity and disability for teachers only adds to the challenges faced by neurodivergent educators like myself. This situation has taken a strain on my emotional and mental well-being, and I always feel like I'm falling short professionally as a result, despite being told by others that what I am experiencing is normal and it is okay to feel how I am feeling. I cannot help but feel incompetent at times, especially when I compare myself to my neuro normative peers who seem to have it more put together than I do and know what they're doing.

I am, however, trying to make some changes for the betterment of disabled and neurodivergent folk. I am firm on trying to incorporate the term 'neurodivergent' when talking about topics 'SEND' related. For instance, during SENCo meetings when talking about the children in my class with EHC Plans, I always make sure I am using the actual term for the neurodivergence such as autism, ADHD, etc. This is my way of normalizing the usage of the terms. Sometimes, when I am able to, I will use the actual word 'neurodivergent' during these meetings when I can. I am fortunate enough to have colleagues who are open to listen and learn about neurodivergence, but there is only so much I can do, however, as I still have to use the term 'SEND' formally when writing up the paperwork as per government guidelines. This is a way for me to unlearn the 'known' and to express a means of change within the workplace in the hopes that it can be normalised as much as how 'SEND' has become normalized and thoughtlessly used. I practice this, what I like to call, 'normalization' of using these terms in any conversation as well with any staff member across the school, and I am always open to talk about my personal experiences to develop an understanding for neurodivergence. I wish term like 'neurodivergence' and 'neuro normativity' as well as actual neurodivergent terms like dyspraxia, ADHD, autism, etc. were normalized, but alas, I do what I can. I also attempt to promote inclusivity instead of conformity by using posters as a tool around my classroom to talk about disability and neurodiversity from the perspective of those in the communities instead of outsiders (i.e. psychiatrists and 'professionals'). I value our voices and firmly believe that they need to 'include' us in any capacity. "Nothing about us without us," in and outside of the classroom.

Independent or non-maintained special schools

These are UK-based specialist educational settings designed specifically for children whose needs cannot be fully met in mainstream or state-funded special schools. They provide tailored teaching methods, specialist staff, and sensory-friendly environments to address students' specific social, emotional, and educational needs. While not governed by local authorities, they may receive funding for Education, Health and Care Plans. Some also offer residential placements for round-the-clock care or when local schools cannot meet a student's requirements. Managed by charitable organisations or private entities, these schools offer alternative pathways where neurodivergent learners can thrive without the constraints of standardised curricula. However, concerns exist around their high costs and inconsistent oversight. Access is also often dependent on parental advocacy and local authority willingness to fund placements, leading to inequities.

Infanticide 🚫

Infanticide refers to the deliberate and deeply troubling act of killing an infant or very young child. It is both morally and legally unacceptable. It often reflects profound societal failures where individuals are driven to unimaginable extremes. The perception that a child may be disabled, including being autistic, can increase the risk of infanticide, especially if compounded by certain socio-cultural factors. One key factor includes societal and cultural stigma around disability, particularly the view in some communities that disabilities are curses or punishments that could lead to social ostracism of the family. Other factors include lack of support for parents, poverty, mental health challenges, and overwhelming social pressures to conform to ideals of cultural 'normalcy.' It is, therefore, an issue that demands careful contextual understanding and often requires us to question societal and cultural structures that lead to such tragic outcomes.

Infantilisation 🚫

Infantilisation is the treatment of autistic adults as if they are children, regardless of their age or abilities. It often involves overly simple language, excessive control over decisions, and assumptions about their capacity to contribute meaningfully. Beyond being patronising, it undermines autonomy, reinforces stereotypes of perpetual dependency, and limits opportunities for growth, self-expression, and inclusion. This issue extends beyond individual interactions, embedding itself in institutional practices, healthcare systems, and societal attitudes. Addressing infantilisation requires treating autistic and neurodivergent people as equal participants, recognising their abilities and needs with respect rather than diminishing them.

Infodumping 💬 👥

An 'infodump' (or 'monologuing') refers to a communication style where an individual, often without realising it, shares a large amount of information on a particular topic all at once. While it can overwhelm listeners, for autistic people, it often reflects deep passion, joy, and engagement with areas of specialised interest, sometimes linked to monotropism. Neurotypical listeners may misinterpret this as excessive or unsocial, leading to misunderstandings in social interactions. The experience can also overwhelm the speaker, who might sense a need to stop but struggle to pause due to being in a focused flow state. Infodumping is not a lack of social awareness but an expression of genuine enthusiasm and connection to a subject.

Inner monologue

An inner monologue refers to the continuous, often complex, flow of thoughts within a person's mind, reflecting self-talk, emotions, or the narrative voice that processes experiences. For many, inner monologue plays a key role in organising their daily lives, decision-making, and reflecting on past events. For neurodivergent individuals, particularly autistic people, an inner monologue can manifest in a vividly descriptive or emotionally charged way, while others may have more visual or sensory forms of internal processing rather than linguistic thought. For instance, memories might replay as visual snapshots, intense emotions, or specific smells, and decision-making may involve mental flowcharts or physical sensations of 'yes' or 'no.' No single style of internal processing is more valid – each reflects the rich diversity of human cognition shaped by individual neurotypes.

Integrated care boards

Integrated care boards (ICBs) were introduced in NHS reforms to unify health and care services across England. There are 42 ICBs, each responsible for allocating budgets, commissioning services, and overseeing performance within their integrated care systems. Their structure includes a chair, CEO, and representatives from NHS providers, general practice, and local authorities.

ICBs aim to integrate health and care sectors, including hospitals, GP services, social care, and mental health services, to reduce fragmentation and address gaps in care. This regional planning focuses on improving service coordination and ensuring tailored support for local populations, including neurodivergent individuals.

However, ICBs face significant challenges. Workforce shortages and inadequate funding have hindered their ability to meet targets. Integration of services like social care and mental health has also been limited, with slow progress on broader health determinants such as housing and employment.

Internalised ableism

Internalised ableism occurs when neurodivergent individuals absorb and adopt the negative stereotypes and prejudices of society about their differences. This can lead to self-criticism, self-doubt, and attempts to conform to neurotypical standards, often at great emotional and psychological cost. Autistic people may suppress their natural traits or mask their identity to be accepted, which can result in depression, heightened anxiety, burnout, a diminished sense of self-worth, and suicidal ideation.

This internal conflict stems from the pervasive societal notion that neurotypical ways of thinking, communicating, and behaving are inherently superior. Exposure to positive autistic role models and engagement with the autistic community can help counteract these negative effects. Additionally, family support, access to safe spaces, and positive peer interactions play crucial roles in how internalised ableism develops, is maintained, or defined. Ultimately, overcoming internalised ableism requires both individual self-acceptance and broader cultural shifts towards valuing all neurological identities as equal.

Interoception

Interoception is the awareness of internal bodily signals, such as hunger, thirst, heartbeat, pain, and toileting needs. Many autistic people experience interoceptive differences, either being hypersensitive or hyposensitive to these signals. This can lead to difficulties recognising thirst, hunger, or pain, potentially delaying responses to health issues and worsening symptoms.

These differences are linked to sensory processing and significantly affect emotional regulation, as internal bodily signals often influence how emotions are felt and managed.

Strategies to support interoception include keeping a daily diary to track meals, hydration, sleep, and physical sensations. Trusted individuals, or 'safe partners,' can help autistic people identify and communicate their internal states, particularly when recognising pain or illness. Technology, such as smartwatches that monitor heart rate, hydration, and sleep patterns, can also provide valuable prompts and insights, improving health management and overall well-being.

Interoceptive alexithymia

Interoceptive alexithymia specifically refers to difficulties in recognising, identifying, or describing emotions that are tied to internal bodily sensations (interoception). Unlike general alexithymia, which encompasses a broader range of challenges in emotional awareness and expression, interoceptive alexithymia focuses on the disconnection between physical sensations and emotional states.

For example, individuals may notice physical signs like an increased heartbeat or muscle tension but struggle to interpret these as anxiety, excitement, or other emotions. This specific difficulty impacts emotional regulation by limiting the ability to link bodily experiences with their emotional meanings, which can make processing, expressing, and managing emotions more challenging.

Intersectionality ⚖️

Intersectionality refers to the interconnected nature of social identities and how they combine to create different modes of discrimination or privilege. The term highlights how people's overlapping identities – such as race, gender, class, disability, and neurology – shape their experiences of oppression. For neurodivergent individuals, intersectionality is a vital concept because it acknowledges that they do not exist in isolation from other social categories. Being autistic and also, for instance, a transgender individual or from a low-income background can result in compounded challenges that are not just additive but fundamentally alter how marginalisation is experienced. Understanding intersectionality within neurodiversity allows for a more nuanced appreciation of each individual's unique experience, emphasising that solutions to inequality must address the intersections of these identities rather than treating them as separate issues.

IN MY OWN WORDS: WILLIAM VANDERPUYE

Prior to the commencement of my social work degree, I came across a book titled *Intersectionality*. It was part of my reading list. I had never heard the term before, and I struggled to understand the concept. Being a bit of a linguist, I explored the etymology of the term. The Latin prefix 'inter' means 'among or in between' and the French surgical term 'séction,' which means 'to cut, to slice or to dissect.' To me, intersectionality therefore meant "how the different portions (or sections) of my identity interact to make me who I am and to make my life what it is. It has determined how people have perceived me, treated me, and it has been a defining factor on how opportunities are created or lost for me."

Kimberlé Crenshaw, an American legal scholar and civil rights advocate, coined the term 'intersectionality' in 1989 to explain and explore the various forms of discriminations that faced individuals, especially black women.

As for my intersectionality, I am a black male, first generation migrant, African, British, dual citizen. I am also Neurodivergeant (AuDHD).

Previously I would reflect on my life, consider my age and compare myself to other people who are younger than me and are a lot more successful,

famous and wealthier than me. I would blame myself for "being a failure" in spite of having a ten or twenty-year head start ahead of them. It is not the colour of their skin, because I would then begin to name successful young black people.

– "but I'm a first generation migrant" I would say to myself, only to remember a handful of first generation black Africans whose renown and contributions have made a measurable impact on society.

"Yeah, but they're not autistic!" I would argue with myself defensively, as my brain parades images of autistic artists, musicians, actors, and authors – some of whom are billionaires and sought-after public speakers. Then I realise that each of them has an aspect of what has been used to discriminate against me. However, not all of them possess ALL of those identities. These identities have amplified the magnitude of discrimination I've faced in life.

Understanding this makes me kinder to myself. I tell myself, "It's not your fault that you haven't achieved what you envisioned as a child, given your intelligence." Yet part of my brain tries to convince me otherwise, that it is my fault, that I haven't worked hard enough. There are people around me who want me to believe this too – that I'm not "making an effort" and that I'm using autism as an excuse.

But for me, understanding intersectionality has been empowering. It has made me feel less depressed and more validated.

Intrusive memories

Intrusive memories are recurrent, involuntary memories of past experiences that can be distressing or overwhelming. They are often linked to traumatic events and can resurface without warning, impacting on daily life. For autistic people, the sensory and emotional intensity of such memories may be heightened, particularly if they are associated with past experiences of sensory overload, social exclusion, or trauma (including PTSD). Monotropic thinking may also lead to more vivid and detailed memory formation, with the individual focusing their attention on the details of these memories particularly intensely.

Intrusive thoughts

Intrusive thoughts are unwanted, involuntary thoughts, images, or ideas that can be distressing and persistent. While common among neurodivergent individuals, including autistic people, they are not exclusive to any neurotype. Intrusive thoughts are often misunderstood; while they can be disturbing, they are rarely reflective of one's true desires or intentions.

Intrusive thoughts become more problematic when they cause significant anxiety or when attempts to suppress them increase their frequency and intensity. Autistic individuals may be especially prone to heightened anxiety from sensory overload, routine changes, or social pressures, amplifying intrusive thoughts. Similarly, those with obsessive-compulsive disorder (OCD) may experience particularly intense intrusive thoughts.

Accepting that these thoughts do not define one's character is essential for managing their impact effectively.

Invisible disability

An invisible disability, also sometimes termed a psychosocial disability, refers to disabilities that are 'unseen' and are less immediately apparent and visible to others. This includes neurological differences like autism and ADHD, physical conditions such as chronic pain and fibromyalgia, and mental health issues like depression.

The hidden nature of these disabilities often leads to misunderstanding, with others failing to recognise or respect the challenges involved. Society may unfairly perceive individuals with invisible disabilities as lazy or exaggerating their struggles, increasing stigma and delaying support.

Support can be improved through inclusive practices, personalised accommodations, and environments that enable understanding, acceptance, and empowerment.

IN MY OWN WORDS: HAZEL LIM

Not all disabilities are visible. Despite outward appearances of success and capability, I've come to understand that 'disability' isn't synonymous with limitation but rather encompasses unique abilities. However, as I've navigated life's journey, I've realised that the coping mechanisms I've employed to persevere have obscured my challenges, classifying them as 'invisible disabilities.' This invisibility often leads to misunderstandings and societal hurdles, exemplified by questions like, "you don't look autistic," which perpetuate this misconception. Many associate autism and neurodivergence with visible conditions, such as using a wheelchair, or with stereotypical

behaviours, which often elicit more empathy and understanding. Nevertheless, my neurodifferences aren't immediately apparent, making it challenging for others to recognise and accommodate my needs.

Mainstream society often overlooks the consideration of neurodiversity in its designs, making it arduous for neurodivergent individuals like me to receive equal understanding and, in turn, feeling 'disabled.' While neurodivergence can indeed be a strength, it also presents challenges that aren't readily comprehended by prevailing societal norms. The built environment and social structures frequently neglect the needs of neurodiverse individuals, leaving us feeling 'disabled' in certain situations.

Moreover, neurodivergent individuals like myself often possess heightened sensitivity to energies, significantly influencing our reactions and abilities. Although energy itself is invisible, its impact is profound, shaping our perceptions and interactions with the world. This sensitivity enables us to discern both positive and negative energies, affecting our daily experiences. For instance, exposure to environments with positive energy can enhance our well-being and productivity, while exposure to negative energy can be overwhelming.

Recognising and respecting this sensitivity to energies within the neurodivergent community is paramount. Establishing inclusive environments that acknowledge and accommodate these sensitivities is essential for fostering understanding and acceptance. By embracing neurodiversity in all its facets, including our sensitivity to energies, we can cultivate a more compassionate and inclusive society where individuals are valued for their unique abilities and experiences. It's time to transcend visible disabilities and acknowledge the diverse ways in which individuals perceive and interact with the world, embracing neurodiversity as an integral aspect of human variation.

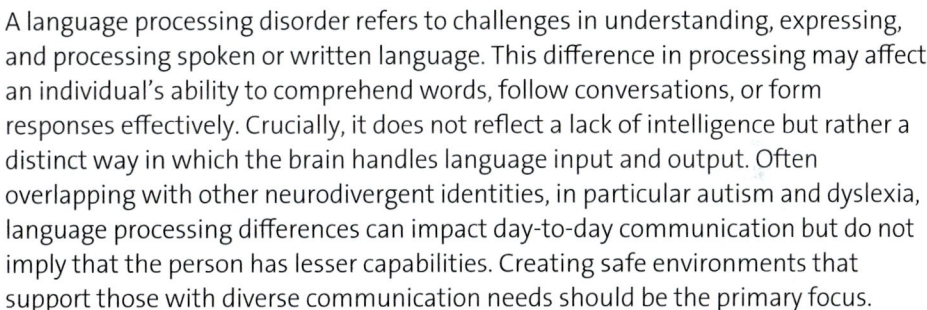

Language processing disorder

A language processing disorder refers to challenges in understanding, expressing, and processing spoken or written language. This difference in processing may affect an individual's ability to comprehend words, follow conversations, or form responses effectively. Crucially, it does not reflect a lack of intelligence but rather a distinct way in which the brain handles language input and output. Often overlapping with other neurodivergent identities, in particular autism and dyslexia, language processing differences can impact day-to-day communication but do not imply that the person has lesser capabilities. Creating safe environments that support those with diverse communication needs should be the primary focus.

Late diagnosis

Late diagnosis refers to formally identifying someone as autistic or neurodivergent later in life, often in adulthood. This delay can result in years of confusion, mental health struggles, and social challenges due to a lack of self-understanding. Barriers to timely diagnosis disproportionately affect women, non-binary people, and non-stereotypically presenting men, reflecting outdated attitudes and systemic flaws in healthcare and society. The risk of late diagnosis is closely tied to the general understanding of autism in a community – the more stigmatised autism is, the more likely a late diagnosis will be.

Despite the challenges, receiving a diagnosis at any age can be profoundly life-affirming, offering clarity and a path towards self-acceptance and empowerment. It can also prompt institutions, such as schools and employers, to provide legally mandated support.

Currently, a diagnosis is considered late if it occurs in an individual's 20s or later. However, as autism acceptance and understanding advance, the threshold for a 'late' diagnosis should shift this threshold to early primary school years. A late diagnosis is similar to 'late identification,' where individuals are recognised as neurodivergent by themselves or others without necessarily having a formal diagnosis.

IN MY OWN WORDS: ANDREW KINGSLOW

I was diagnosed in my mid-40s. Life had become unbearable, as years of masking had taken their toll on me. My anxiety, meltdowns, burnout, and depression cycles had started to rule my life. Pre-diagnosis, I had developed many analogies to explain away my behaviours – "I'm like a shark because I can't breathe if I'm not moving," or "There are only two states in life: bored or scared. I'd rather spend my life scared." I had constantly failed at relationships due to a lack of emotional connection.

What eventually pushed me into actively masking was bullying – not just from peers but from teachers too. I was often singled out, cajoled, and removed from class for not sharing common opinions or for being obtrusive in my questioning.

From an academic perspective, I had scored very highly on IQ tests and was therefore pushed up a year and given a private tutor for maths, etc. I'd hide under the bed when my mum was vacuuming because the noise was so deafening. I had perfect pitch. Does all of this sound familiar or stereotypical?

I can honestly say, with hand on heart, that as a child I felt different. I didn't want to follow the same path as others and felt outside the norm, like being 'normal' wouldn't satisfy my needs.

The core of all these experiences led to one thing: being on the outside. Every interaction was based on what I thought I should be rather than what I actually was. The constant second-guessing led to much anxiety, and years of learned survival techniques left me exhausted.

Of course, people had joked about me being autistic at various times, and I guess deep down I knew it was a possibility. But what diagnosis gave me was the opportunity to get support and finally unpack all the layers I had built up over the years.

I look at late diagnosis as a form of grief; it follows most of the classic stages: denial, anger, depression, and acceptance.

Denial (or Imposter Syndrome): It can't be true because I'm too normal, and I've functioned my whole life just fine up until now. (Of course, I haven't functioned fine, which is why I'm still single with no children, riddled with PDA, and just terrible at dealing with day-to-day life).

Anger: I'm so angry at those who bullied me, those who didn't understand, those who made fun, those who took advantage, and mostly at myself for not showing compassion when it was needed.

Depression: I messed my life up. Everything could have been different had I been diagnosed earlier. How will I cope with this life now? I feel pathologised and utterly exhausted having to function in a world that is now confusing and illogical.

Acceptance: Primarily acceptance of help as well as accepting that I can only control my reaction to life and not life itself.

With late diagnosis comes the absolute need for therapy that caters specifically to the individual's neuro-identity, whether that's Autism, ADHD, or AuDHD. In my case, my logical brain has benefitted hugely from being given actual reasons for my patterned behaviour from a clinical point of view. This has, in turn, allowed me to be kind to myself in certain situations and work through some of my addictive traits in a much more measured and informed way.

Late diagnosis comes with many downsides, but I'd choose it a thousand times over no diagnosis.

Learning disabilities and learning difficulties 💬 🏢

Learning disabilities refer to significant, lifelong impairments in intellectual ability (as defined by predominant neurotypical perspectives on intelligence), impacting upon a broad range of life skills, including learning, communication, and self-care. These disabilities often result in difficulties with learning and understanding new information, extending beyond academic performance.

In contrast, learning difficulties are specific to challenges in academic areas like reading, writing, or mathematics, without affecting overall intellectual ability. Known as specific learning difficulties (SpLDs), these include dyslexia (reading), dyscalculia (mathematics), and dysgraphia (writing). Individuals with learning difficulties often excel in other areas and develop effective strategies to navigate their challenges.

It is important to recognise both groups can thrive with the right support, tools, and understanding. Recognising diverse learning styles and adapting traditional education systems are essential to ensure inclusivity and equity for all learners.

Legal advocacy ⚖️

Legal advocacy for neurodivergent people focuses on protecting their rights and ensuring fair treatment within legal systems. It addresses discrimination, promotes equal access to services, and pushes for inclusive legal procedures that respect neurodivergent needs. Advocates work to ensure fair representation in courts, education, and workplaces, challenging pressures to conform to neurotypical norms and opposing coercive practices like autistic masking or harmful therapies.

Legal advocacy is a critical tool in dismantling structural ableism and ensuring that neurodivergent people are treated with dignity and respect, particularly in environments that are often hostile or exclusionary to difference.

Letter-boarding 💬 👥

Letter-boarding is a communication method used by non-speaking autistic people, involving pointing to or selecting letters on a board to spell out words. It enables individuals to express complex thoughts, challenging misconceptions about their cognitive abilities and emphasising that speech is not the sole form of meaningful communication.

This method provides an accessible way to engage with others and empowers non-speaking autistic individuals by offering an alternative communication tool tailored to their needs. However, its use must always remain voluntary, ensuring it does not become a source of coercion or stress.

Literal thinking 💬

Literal thinking is a cognitive style where words and concepts are interpreted in their most direct sense, without relying on implied or metaphorical meanings. This form of thinking can be common among autistic people as it reflects a preference for clear, unambiguous communication.

While neurotypical individuals often navigate idioms, sarcasm, and nuance with ease, these forms of language can feel confusing or misleading to literal thinkers. This preference for literal language aligns with the broader concept of the 'double empathy problem,' which highlights the mutual misunderstandings that can occur between autistic and non-autistic people. Embracing literal thinking can enhance communication by reducing ambiguity, ultimately enabling better understanding between diverse neurotypes.

IN MY OWN WORDS: KOSJENKA PETEK

"Gosh, mum, you're soooo autistic. How can you live like that?!"

This is something I hear from my autistic teenager quite often – usually whenever my literal thinking slips into our conversations, which is daily.

Am I the family's laughing stock because of my literal thinking? Yes, I am. And while it doesn't bother me as much now, it used to. It made me feel small, inadequate, and flawed – until I went through my autism assessment. My literal thinking even makes me the life of the party, or at least the in-house clown. It's not unlike how I was during my school days. Sound familiar? I sometimes think stand-up comedy might just be my calling.

My friends often tell me they enjoy my company because I take things at face value, and we share so many laughs when I comment on what I've *actually* heard them say. I love laughing with my friends and making them laugh. It's different with them – they laugh *with* me, not *at* me. With people who truly love, like, and accept you for who you are, you don't have to worry about being misunderstood. They don't question your intelligence, sincerity, intentions, or work ethic. You can simply be yourself.

But everything changes when I leave the safety of home or the company of loving friends.

Literal thinking means I don't always catch the hidden messages people often embed in their words. Social communication and interaction are my biggest autism challenges. When I think about navigating the outside world as a literal thinker, I feel an overwhelming grief – deep, consuming, and suffocating. It makes me feel small, inadequate, and even stupid. Over the years, I've been labelled as unintelligent because of my literal thinking. Bullies at various jobs targeted me for my inability to convey or understand subtext. Too often, people added meanings to my words or actions that simply weren't there.

And it's not just non-autistic people. Even neurodivergent individuals with stronger social skills have misunderstood me and, at times, bullied me too. What I've come to realise is that my literal thinking confuses both non-autistic and autistic people alike. Subtext is power, and no one seems entirely immune to its grip.

It has taken me a long time to embrace my literal thinking and shed the shame I felt about my inability to read between the lines. It's still a work in progress, but now I know I'm not illiterate or cognitively impaired. My autism diagnostician explained this to me kindly, and it helped more than I can say.

There are good days and bad days. I'm often petrified of making a mistake in communication, of missing a subtextual cue, or of unintentionally hurting someone. This fear can trigger a trauma response. I've had to train myself to stay mindful of the fact that I might not fully grasp every layer of a conversation. I've learned to ask a lot of clarifying questions to ensure I understand what's being said.

I also make an effort to check that I've communicated my own thoughts clearly. It's exhausting. It's scary. And yes, it hurts.

Over time, I've developed strategies: I repeat my thoughts during conversations, explain my thought process multiple times, and try to ensure that others understand me well enough to avoid misinterpreting my words. Yet even with these efforts, I often feel like there's no winning. Here's how the cycle typically plays out: my words are misunderstood, some unspoken subtext is ascribed to them, and no one tells me directly. Instead, I'll find out later – through a third party or sometimes after weeks, months, or even years – when someone finally reveals they were hurt or confused by the supposed subtext. When I try to explain myself, I'm often met with a dismissive tone: "You're just justifying your actions again. Like you always do."

Sound familiar? It's not just a non-autistic thing – it's a shared human challenge. The double empathy problem, or even a triple empathy problem, as I see it.

Oh well.

Over time, I've come to accept that many emotionally challenging experiences in my life are tied to being a literal thinker. It's a bittersweet part of my autism. But as I sit here writing this, I can hear my friends' laughter and delight in my mind, and it brings a smile to my face!

Loneliness

For many autistic people, loneliness is not about a desire for isolation, as is often assumed, but rather about the difficulties in finding environments that promote genuine acceptance and understanding. Autistic individuals can and do wish to form deep, meaningful relationships, but they often face social exclusion due to differences in communication styles, sensory sensitivities, or social stigma. Mismatched expectations between neurotypical and neurodivergent interaction styles further reinforce these barriers.

It is also important to distinguish loneliness from aloneness. No one, including autistic and other neurodivergent people, desires loneliness. However, there are times when aloneness is necessary, for self-regulation, especially during anxiety or sensory overwhelm.

Loneliness is commonly understood through two primary types: emotional loneliness, the absence of close, meaningful connections, and social loneliness, a lack of broader social networks or community engagement. Autistic people are particularly vulnerable to both when environments fail to accommodate neurodivergent ways of being.

Addressing loneliness goes beyond providing social opportunities – it requires creating spaces that offer genuine acceptance, understanding, and inclusion for neurodivergent individuals.

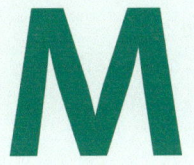

Mainstream schools with SEN support

Mainstream schools with special educational needs (SEN) support refer to educational institutions that primarily cater to the general mainstream student population while also providing tailored assistance for SEN students. This model integrates SEN students into mainstream classrooms, enabling them to learn alongside their peers. Inclusive environments also benefit mainstream students, leading to mutual understanding and respect.

SEN support involves adjustments to teaching methods, classroom environments, and assessments to address diverse needs. The approach emphasises equity, diversity, and inclusion, ensuring all students access a supportive education without segregation. However, the well-intentioned aims of these schools must be backed by real action and a commitment to best practices and high-quality evidence. Teachers' self-efficacy and attitudes towards inclusion also significantly impact the success of inclusive educational practices. As such, effective implementation requires more than just words; it demands dedicated resources, ongoing training, and an unwavering commitment to inclusivity.

IN MY OWN WORDS: KOSJENKA PETEK

Since Croatia began its journey towards EU membership and the adoption of broader European standards in education and social inclusion, the country has been striving to implement inclusive education and policies.

Despite positive reports, we, as autistic teachers, researchers, and inclusion professionals, know all too well that much of Europe grapples with similar challenges in applying inclusive practices. My literal thinking once led me to believe that the Acts and Laws were being followed from the moment they were signed. But over time, I came to realise that these documents were often just symbolic – what we in Croatian call "a dead letter on a piece of paper."

DOI: 10.4324/9781003477297-11

Although the Croatian government signed these agreements, the implementation of Special Educational Needs (SEN) inclusion has been neither timely nor well-prepared. For more than 25 years, the system has been precariously hanging by a thread – a thread that is now snapping. A favourite Croatian saying, *"Who lives, who dies,"* comes to mind, reflecting the grim reality: we might not live to see true inclusion in action. Yet we persist.

Croatia is a unique case. Home education is banned – it is outright illegal. This, combined with the absence of specialist SEN settings for primary-aged students without intellectual disabilities, creates a nightmare for parents. These children are forced into mainstream schools because there is no other option. They are deemed too advanced for specialist schools catering to children with higher support needs but lack the appropriate support in mainstream settings.

Despite this bleak situation, we see opportunities to improve education for all – autistic children, their parents, teachers, SEN provisions in schools, and management alike. Together with a network of allies, autism professionals, and support from autistic advocates across borders, we work tirelessly. As the saying goes, *"Hope is the power of being cheerful in circumstances we know to be desperate."* It's hard work, but I trust the process because without hope, life would be unbearable.

To borrow from Ursula K. Le Guin, I didn't want to leave Omelas, but neither could I accept its illusion of utopia. Instead, like the characters in N.K. Jemisin's *The Ones Who Stay and Fight*, I chose to stay and resist. We've laid the first tile on this road, though the path ahead is far from built. This is a marathon, and we're preparing for the long run.

When I envision the future of education, I see community, love, and hope. I imagine clusters of learning environments open to all children – wheelchair users, the Deaf, the Autistic, the Non-Speakers, children with Down syndrome, and those without disabilities. Together, all of them, learning side by side with their teachers. I picture laughter, mischief, learning, and strong, trusting relationships. To achieve this vision, we must dismantle the current system, not simply repurpose the flawed tools we've inherited.

We must nurture the next generation – the children who will dismantle these systems and build something better. I believe in them because I see them, teach them, listen to them, and love them for who they are. They are fluid, flexible, and authentic free thinkers. We must protect their innate gifts and help them flourish.

> The future already belongs to them. In fact, the future is here. To borrow from William Gibson, the future may seem unevenly distributed, or perhaps it hasn't yet materialised. To bring it into being, we need a transition period – a time to imagine, design, and lead multiple processes at once, with a clear vision of an accessible and inclusive world. My hope for humanity's inclusive future remains steadfast. I believe we can achieve this.

Masking

'Masking', also referred to as camouflaging, refers to the adaptive strategies that autistic and other neurodivergent people often employ, both consciously and subconsciously, to conform to neurotypical social norms. This phenomenon involves the suppression of natural autistic cognition and behaviours, such as stimming, and the adoption of behaviours deemed acceptable by society, such as forced eye contact and mirroring the body language of others. While sometimes a conscious decision, masking can also occur without awareness, only realised when effects like autistic burnout emerge, prompting reflection on the unintended suppression of one's authentic self.

Masking can be driven by the desire to avoid stigma or negative social consequences, but it comes at a significant personal cost. The constant effort to appear neurotypical can lead to increased stress, exhaustion, burnout, and a loss of personal identity, potentially creating and exacerbating mental health problems including suicidal ideation. Women and non-binary individuals may mask their autistic traits particularly effectively, often leading to missed diagnoses. However, all genders are susceptible to masking, and many men likely experience missed or delayed identification of autism due to their own masking behaviours.

The need for masking underscores the pervasive influence of societal expectations that undervalue autistic ways of being. Advocating for environments that celebrate rather than suppress neurodivergent identities is essential for enabling true acceptance and mitigating the harmful impacts of masking.

IN MY OWN WORDS: GINNY GRANT

My mask has taken me 44 years to craft – the exact number of years I have been alive. From a young age, I learned to cover up the traits in me that diverged from the neurotypical norm. I didn't know these as Autistic traits, only as things about me that were different and, possibly, socially unacceptable. As a young child, I learned to hide my anxiety about a world that was all too often alarming to me. As a preteen, I learned to suppress my need to move my body in certain ways, adopting less visible, more socially acceptable habits, such as biting on my hair and lips, scratching at my scalp, tearing at my nails, chewing on pencils and pens, doodling in class. As a teen, I copied the phrasing and behaviours of others around me, and my parents taught me that I needed to make eye contact during conversations, even if it was uncomfortable. I also learned that if I put my hand up for every opportunity at school and beyond, I was more likely to be included socially. And so I went into the world as a young adult, unidentified as Autistic and unsupported. It didn't take long — one year in the adult world — for things to fall apart. I was first diagnosed with depression — Autistic burnout? — at the age of 19.

Since I was formally identified as Autistic, at the age of 39 years, I have become more aware of the traits that non-autistic people see in me, the ways in which I diverge from the norm. According to the clinician in my diagnostic report, I am 'blunt' and 'frank,' and my eye contact is 'overly intense' or 'not there' (you can't win!). It was a blow to my ego to discover that others might think these things about me and, often in social situations, I now find my inner voice questioning whether I am being 'blunt,' 'frank,' or my eye contact is wrong in some way. So I often try to rein in the blunt statements, the frank honesty, the long gaze as part of my mask.

But also since my formal identification as Autistic, I have learned the value of spending time in Autistic space and have enjoyed numerous opportunities, in catch-ups with neurodivergent friends, at retreats and conferences, where I can lower my mask and just be myself — Autistic traits and all. This might look like using stim toys, cuddling weighted toys, relaxing on beanbags, using adaptive technology such as sunglasses, ear buds, or noise-cancelling headphones, not forcing myself to look others in the eye, and saying more or less what I damn well please, without the worry of being 'too blunt,' 'too frank'.

Mate crime 🚫

Mate crime refers to a specific form of exploitation or abuse where someone close to a neurodivergent person — such as a friend, carer, or family member — manipulates or mistreats them under the guise of friendship. Unlike typical hate crimes, perpetrators are often trusted individuals who manipulate their victims for personal gain through cruelty, theft, or humiliation. This may include pressuring them to lend money, commit crimes, or engage in risky behaviours.

Autistic individuals, particularly those who are AuDHD (autistic and ADHD), may struggle to recognise manipulation due to differences in social understanding, heightened trust, or a strong desire for connection. Difficulty managing emotions and actions in the moment can also increase vulnerability.

The emotional fallout from these crimes can be severe, often leading to deep mistrust, anxiety, and depression. Shame or embarrassment about being exploited may prevent individuals from seeking help. Raising awareness about mate crime is essential to protect socially vulnerable people from such harm.

Media representation

Historically, media representation of neurodivergent individuals has been fraught with misrepresentation and stereotypes. For example, the characterisation of autistic individuals as savants, like in the film *Rain Man*, led to the stereotype that all autistic people possess extraordinary abilities, overshadowing the diverse experiences of the autistic community. These portrayals have contributed to lasting stigma, misunderstanding, and discrimination.

More recently, neurodivergent coding has become common, where characters exhibit neurodivergent traits without explicit identification. This trend risks reducing these traits to superficial quirks rather than meaningful representation.

Authentic portrayals require collaboration with neurodivergent individuals throughout the creative process, from concept to final production. This ensures stories are accurate, respectful, and reflective of lived experiences.

Effective representation holds the power to reshape societal attitudes and improve public understanding. Media – whether traditional, social, or digital – bears an ongoing moral responsibility to approach neurodivergent narratives with care and integrity.

IN MY OWN WORDS: IQRA BABAR

The state of neurodivergent media representation fluctuates. Historically, it has always favoured a homogenous depiction of autistic folk and, for the most part, has been incredibly harmful in people's perceptions of us. This includes my perception of myself and how I formerly perceived neurodivergence and disability. Growing up, I strived for 'normality,' whatever that means. I guess the best way I understand it today is the capitalist, corporate external perception of what we as people should be like. This encompasses behaviours, mannerisms, and social cues, amongst other characteristics. Quite frankly, it is

hard. And the media depicting us as a certain way of 'being' in comparison to a 'being' that is framed as 'normal' is toxic and damaging. It directly feeds into creating a warped perception of how people THINK we are instead of understanding how we ACTUALLY are.

Often, the progress of representation in the media is slow. It is even slower to acknowledge and normalise the intersectionality of humans. The level of representation also seems to stop at the White lens. This is what is normalised, instead of showcasing the rich nuances and diversity of the autistic community. We are as diverse as our traits, but it seems as though neurodivergent folk such as myself are left out of the bigger picture to paint an 'idealized' caricature of autism, ADHD, or any other neurodivergency.

One of the most significantly raw and authentic pieces of media representation I have experienced is in the Pixar short film *Loop*. *Loop* follows the main character, Renee, a non-speaking autistic girl, and a chatty boy, who are stuck on a canoeing boat and find ways to communicate with each other. There are barely any words in the short film, but it still succeeds in portraying a raw sensory experience. We explore Renee's communication through her other senses across the lake in a beautifully personal way. The voice actress of Renee is also a non-speaking autistic woman, and the character is visibly a woman of colour. It was captivating, enchanting and real. It was so raw which added to its captivation. The sheer movement of the characters, the seamless interactions, and the realness of it all felt so rewarding to watch.

Often, characters with autism are portrayed using stereotypes because the creators don't bother to do proper research. For example, Shaun from *The Good Doctor* and Sheldon Cooper in *The Big Bang Theory* are caricatures that, unfortunately, present as the faces of 'autistic representation.' That's not to say that there are not people out there who will resonate with them, but their caricatures should not be the standard, nor should they be used as a justification to continue portraying these caricatures. I, for instance, cannot stand these two portrayals, especially because they are not played by autistics themselves, but by neuro-normative men instead. It feels inauthentic and lazy to me. It is also problematic that what people perceive as the epitome of autistic media representation are White-male caricatures and nothing outside of that binary.

Due to disparities in media representation of autistic individuals and neurodivergence in general, many people from these communities have developed 'headcanons,' for existing characters that they believe to be autistic, ADHD, or any other neurodivergent identity. A 'headcanon' is a fan interpretation of a character or a story. For example, some fans interpret Kamala Khan from Marvel Comics as having ADHD, Lilo from *Lilo and Stitch* as autistic, and Sailor Moon as dyspraxic. A few years ago, I created an online thread discussing the possibility of Kamala Khan, a.k.a. Ms Marvel, having ADHD. The thread gained a lot of attention, and to this day, I still receive interactions on it. It brings me joy to know that many others share my perspective on her character and how she has been portrayed. This validation of my view, especially as an ADHDer, feels fulfilling. Additionally, it's allowed me to connect with like-minded individuals, particularly those in the neurodivergent community, forming a sense of unity and liberation within these spaces.

The absence of diverse representation beyond the White-male binary led to the emergence of the hashtag #nothingaboutuswithoutus. This movement seeks to involve autistic individuals in the creation of content related to autism, including characters and stories; the same principle applies to other neurodivergent identities. As someone who didn't see people like myself represented in the media growing up, I fully support and contribute to this movement. It is pivotal to centre intersectional voices, it is not enough to just include them. In my case, Peter Parker, a.k.a Spiderman, who looked nothing like me and didn't reflect that side of my identity, was the closest representation I had. I have always longed for characters who not only acted like me but also looked like me. Embracing intersectionality, I am optimistic that the growing presence of neurodivergent creators will lead to better media representation and rise in the ranks of Hollywood and mainstream media.

IN MY OWN WORDS: ADITI GANGRADE

I've always loved watching films and TV shows. For me, they've been a way to cope, dissociate, and decompress.

Growing up in Tier-2 cities in India as a Gen Z kid, I was surrounded by people who adored Indian cinema. Actors were seen as idols, and movies had a lasting impact on people. It wasn't uncommon for someone to mimic a character they loved, adopting their mannerisms, catchphrases, and even their values.

But even though I enjoyed the films I watched, I never truly related to the characters on screen.

Most Bollywood characters felt worlds apart from my reality.

Even during times when Indian cinema was making efforts to show diversity – sometimes veering into stereotypes – I never saw an authentic portrayal of an autistic character. In fact, it was rare to see anyone with visible or invisible disabilities in films, TV shows, or ads.

For the longest time, I thought everyone was the same – that we all came into this world with the same kind of mind and body.

It wasn't until later that I realized this wasn't true. And when I did, I became painfully aware of the biases and stigma surrounding autism: that Autistic people can't work, get married, live independently, or lead full lives.

It felt like autistic people were invisible, as if we only existed behind closed doors or in 'mental hospitals.'

Looking back, I now understand why no one wanted to be friends with the kids who were different – who communicated differently or had needs that others couldn't understand like the need to stim or move around constantly or the need for a quiet space.

My uncle, who lived with multiple disabilities including autism, was treated like he was 'defective' all his life.

Nobody in my family took the effort to learn Indian Sign Language or understand why my uncle had meltdowns. He was labeled difficult and thankless (for not being grateful to the family that fed him and gave him a shelter despite him being disabled). This sounds awful and makes me livid just thinking about it.

My uncle was left out of almost all conversations. He could only communicate about his basic needs including food, water, and wanting to go out. Elders in my family never gave him agency to have a full life – to do a job, get married, communicate how he felt, take decisions for the family, or even discuss his mental health.

Disability wasn't even an afterthought for most people around me. In their eyes, a disabled person's only future was begging on the streets.

Terms like autism, Down syndrome, dyslexia, and mental illness were so stigmatized that most people just used "mental" or "pagal" (Hindi for crazy) to talk about anyone who didn't fit their definition of "normal."

The media I consumed often reinforced these harmful stereotypes, spreading misinformation and perpetuating biases.

Many Indian films mocked disabilities, and they still do. People use the scenes from these films to make memes mocking neurodivergence – disabling humour.

Growing up, I always felt out of place, mostly because I never felt seen or heard by the media I consumed.

But thankfully, things have evolved. Today, we see more media representation in films, shows, ads, and digital content.

For me, good media representation means seeing an autistic character written by autistic writers and played by an autistic actor. As an Autistic ADHD filmmaker, I've witnessed firsthand the power that lived experience brings to a story and a character.

I've said it over and over again: We need autistic filmmakers not just for better autistic representation but because it allows the world, for once, to see life through our eyes.

My mantra to good neurodiversity representation in media – C.L.A.R.I.T.Y

> Challenge – Does it challenge societal biases, stereotypes, and neuronormativity?
>
> Language – Is the language disability affirming and respectful?
>
> Authenticity – Does It have neurodivergent people in the cast or crew? Are the characters complex and layered without simplifying or generalizing neurodivergence?
>
> Realism – Is it realistic? Does it account for neurodivergent lived experience? (without sensationalizing, demonizing, or romanticizing neurodivergence)
>
> Impact – What impact does it have on neurodivergent people?
>
> Tokenism – Does it use neurodivergence as a quirky trait? Does it seem like a checkbox activity? Does the character have a meaningful role and relationships? Do the characters have a purpose beyond their neurodivergent traits?
>
> You – How did you feel watching it?

In the many short documentaries I've directed, we've profiled neurodivergent and disabled individuals. And I strongly feel representation in nonfiction is just as important.

I make it a point to speak to our protagonists well in advance, to hear their stories and understand their perspectives. As a director, my priority is to ensure they feel comfortable and safe sharing their truth.

Our filmmaking processes are neurodiversity-affirming, LGBTQIA-affirming, and trauma-informed. We seek consent at every stage, tailor our methods for non-speaking autistic individuals, and create an environment where people can openly express their needs.

Our goal is to make films that allow marginalized voices to be seen and heard while breaking down stigma in the most positive and authentic way possible.

If young Aditi had seen autistic representation on screen, she might have been bolder, more vocal about her needs, and a lot less prone to feeling like an imposter.

Good representation has the power to change lives. It's time society starts unlearning and relearning the way it sees disability.

Mediation

Mediation for neurodivergent individuals refers to a structured process aimed at resolving disputes or misunderstandings. This may occur in settings where neurodivergent and neurotypical communication styles differ and misunderstanding has occurred, resulting in a potential conflict. Mediation supports all parties to work collaboratively, ensuring that neurodivergent voices are heard and respected, and it can be used in various situations such as workplace conflicts, educational disagreements, or healthcare settings. The aim is to create an environment of acceptance and inclusion, promoting equality and respect for neurodivergent individuals.

Medical model of disability

The medical model of disability is a framework that views disability as an individual problem or deficit that resides within the person, often focusing on medical diagnosis and treatment. This model suggests that to 'fix' or 'cure' the disabled individual, interventions should aim to bring them closer to what is considered 'normal' functioning. In this paradigm, there is a strong emphasis on impairments being inherently negative and in need of medical or therapeutic correction.

On the other hand, the social model of disability positions the socio-cultural environment as the disabling factor. It advocates for societal and structural changes to reduce barriers rather than focusing on altering the individual. The medical model's focus on pathology often ignores the value of neurodiversity and the importance of acceptance.

Meerkat mode

Meerkat mode refers to a heightened state of sensory vigilance experienced by autistic people when they feel unsafe, overwhelmed, or anxious. In this state, an individual may exhibit hyper-awareness, vigilantly scanning their surroundings in an attempt to identify and mitigate potential threats. 'Meerkating' can be triggered by various stressors, including unpredictable environments, unfamiliar social interactions, felt stigma, or sensory overload, which can be especially intense for autistic people, in part, due to their unique sensory processing.

Although the term evokes the image of a meerkat standing upright, alert to danger, this state reflects the profound need for safety and control, not paranoia or irrational fear. Meerkat mode can be exhausting, as it involves sustained attention and heightened anxiety.

Meltdown   🚫

A meltdown is an intense response to overwhelming sensory or emotional input that neurodivergent people, especially autistic individuals, may experience. It is not a behavioural choice but a neurological and psychological reaction to being overstimulated or overwhelmed. Triggers often include sensory overload, frustration, or sudden changes in routine, with the onset varying from rapid escalation to a gradual build-up. This concept aligns with spoon theory, where a meltdown may occur when an autistic person exhausts their limited energy reserves, or 'spoons.'

During a meltdown, an individual might cry, yell, or shut down entirely. This may be incorrectly perceived by others as a tantrum, which instead are deliberate outbursts aimed at achieving a goal. Unfortunately, this difference is often misunderstood, leading to meltdowns being stigmatised as 'bad behaviour' or intentional, much like tantrums may be. It should be recognised that after a meltdown, the person understands they did not have a tantrum, as this mislabelling can increase internalised ableism.

Supporting meltdowns should prioritise understanding rather than punishment. Interruptions should be avoided unless safety is at risk. Calm, predictable, sensory-appropriate, and low-demand environments can help reduce both the frequency and intensity of meltdowns. Recognising meltdowns as expressions of overwhelm rather than deliberate defiance is key to offering meaningful support.

Mental Capacity Act 2005 ⚖️

The Mental Capacity Act 2005 provides a legal framework in England and Wales for decision-making on behalf of individuals aged 16 and over who are unable to make certain decisions themselves, often described as 'lacking capacity.' It covers financial, medical, and personal welfare decisions and emphasises supporting individuals to make their own choices wherever possible. Actions taken on their behalf must prioritise their best interests while respecting their rights and freedoms. Safeguards, such as the Independent Mental Capacity Advocate, were introduced to ensure representation for individuals without family or friends in serious decisions.

Despite its intentions, the Act has faced criticism, particularly regarding how capacity is assessed and its principles applied in practice. The definition of capacity can be overly rigid, failing to account for how neurodivergent individuals, including autistic people, might struggle with communication or decision-making in ways that do not reflect an actual lack of capacity. Assessors may overlook these nuances, leading to inappropriate conclusions about someone's ability to manage their affairs. The 'best interest' principle has also been criticised for inconsistent interpretation, with decisions sometimes reflecting professional biases rather than the individual's preferences.

In 2019, the Mental Capacity (Amendment) Act introduced the Liberty Protection Safeguards to streamline the authorisation of liberty restrictions where necessary. However, implementation has been slow, and concerns persist about the potential for these safeguards to impose excessive restrictions on neurodivergent individuals if applied without care and sensitivity.

IN MY OWN WORDS: WILLIAM VANDERPUYE

Part of my duties as a social worker is to conduct mental capacity assessments to establish whether or not a client has the capacity to make decisions around their health and support needs, their finances, or about where they would like to live following their discharge from hospital. The focus of the assessment is on the decision to be made and every effort is made to empower the client to communicate, either with words, gestures, facial expressions, in writing, or with signs. Additionally, I would arrange for an interpreter if English is not the client's first language. A client may wish to be supported by a friend or a family member or an advocate.

The capacity assessment essentially seeks to establish if the client has the mental capacity to make decisions at that time. It is made up of two parts: the diagnostic test and the functional test. The diagnostic test establishes whether or not the client has a condition or impairment of the mind or their brain resulting from an ailment or usage of a substance. The functional test seeks to establish whether the individual can understand the information, remember the information long enough to make the decision, communicate their wishes and their decision in any possible way, and weigh up the information and the risks of making that decision.

Reflecting on this practice in the context of the Mental Capacity Act 2005, I am reminded of how far we've come since the time and place where I grew up. Back then, people with disabilities did not have the rights and privileges they have today. People with impairments of the mind were treated with a lot less dignity and decisions were made for them by others without including them in the decision-making process. It is of utmost importance to include the subject of the decision in the decision-making process because they will be affected primarily by that decision. So, I like the way every possible means is employed to include the person in the decision-making process or at least to get their views. This reminds me of the saying in the autistic community "Nothing about us without us."

I also think the Act is, in itself, an anti-oppressive measure because it prevents multiple exploitations of the individual by friends, family, and professionals by assisting the decision-making around finances, relationships, healthcare, and more.

Mental Health Act 1983

The Mental Health Act 1983 governs the treatment and rights of individuals in England and Wales who are detained ('sectioned') in hospital settings due to mental health needs. It provides a legal framework for assessment, care, and treatment without consent when necessary. Despite its intentions, the Act has faced criticism for its use with autistic people and those with learning disabilities, often inappropriately.

In England, around 65% of autistic individuals and people with learning disabilities in mental health units are detained under this Act. Many do not have co-occurring mental health conditions but are admitted during crises linked to inadequate community support. These settings frequently fail to meet their needs, with sensory challenges and unsuitable care worsening distress. This often leads to extended stays and harmful practices such as overmedication, restraint, and seclusion.

In 2024, the UK government introduced a Mental Health Bill to reform the Act. Proposed changes include limiting the detention of autistic individuals and those with learning disabilities who do not have co-occurring mental health conditions to a maximum of 28 days. The bill also seeks to mandate personalised care plans and increase the frequency of clinical reviews to ensure appropriate and timely care. While these reforms represent progress, they are still going through the legislative process and have not yet become law.

Mimicry

Mimicry refers to the act of adopting behaviours, mannerisms, or communication styles typically associated with non-autistic people in order to blend in or avoid negative reactions. This form of adaptive morphing, often driven by societal pressure to conform to neurotypical norms, can place a significant mental and emotional strain on autistic individuals as well as identity confusion and exhaustion, potentially contributing to autistic burnout. The act of mimicking is not an expression of one's natural self but rather a survival strategy used to navigate social situations that are unsupportive of neurodivergence. Over time, frequent reliance on mimicry can contribute to issues like anxiety and burnout, as it forces individuals to suppress their authentic ways of thinking and interacting with the world.

Minimally speaking people

The term 'minimally speaking people' refers to autistic individuals who communicate using few spoken words, but this does not equate to an inherent inability to express themselves. Instead, these people often rely on alternative communication methods such as augmentative and alternative communication (AAC), gestures, body language, or written text. While their verbal speech may be limited, their capacity for complex thought and communication is not diminished. It is important to reject assumptions that minimising verbal communication correlates with cognitive ability or understanding, as such views perpetuate harmful stereotypes.

Minority and intersectional minority stress

Minority stress describes the unique and additional stress experienced by individuals from marginalised groups due to systemic inequities, societal stigma, and a lack of acceptance. For neurodivergent people, this stress often stems from pressures to conform to neurotypical norms and the pervasive effects of ableism. When neurodivergence intersects with other marginalised identities, such as ethnicity, gender, or LGBTQ+ status, the resulting intersectional minority stress creates additional layers of discrimination and exclusion.

For example, imagine a Black, non-binary autistic teenager navigating their school environment. They face implicit racial biases that label their self-advocacy as defiance, gender norms that invalidate their identity, and ableist attitudes that dismiss their neurodivergent identity. During a class discussion about emotions, a teacher may dismiss their input, assuming they will not be able to understand it. A peer mocks their voice and mannerisms. They report the incident, but the school counsellor, failing to understand their intersectional identity, suggests they 'try to fit in more.' The teenager is left feeling unheard, unseen, and overwhelmed, grappling with the cumulative weight of racism, gender discrimination, and ableism.

This daily reality not only impacts their mental health but also sends a deeper message: they are expected to erase parts of who they are to be accepted. The emotional toll of constantly battling societal structures designed without their needs in mind becomes a quiet, lingering burden.

IN MY OWN WORDS: KOSJENKA PETEK

I am not an angry autistic.

Not anymore.

It has taken me six years since my official diagnosis to stand here and say these words.

I *was* an angry autistic.

When the very core of your being is stigmatised, discriminated against, mocked, or rejected, it's a heavy burden to carry from the moment you step into the world. Members of my family, kindergarten teachers, primary and secondary school teachers, romantic partners, and even friends – so many of them – disliked, chastised, or worked hard to show me I wasn't a 'normal' human being. Little did they know I hadn't felt 'normal' since I was five or six years old. Back then, I was convinced aliens had left me here and that one day, my mothership would come back for me. *Hurry up, Mothership, please!*

But the mothership never came. The discrimination and stigmatisation of how I exist and move through the human world continued.

When my autism diagnostician explained that the things labelled *wrong* about me were perfectly normal for someone on the autism spectrum (or, as she said, for a woman with Asperger's syndrome), I was consumed by anger. So much anger! It wasn't just mine – it was the collective anger of many other autistic women, queer autistic women, all of us carrying the weight of minority stress. At some point, that stress overflowed into self-advocacy, public advocacy, and our interactions with autism professionals.

When we founded the ASK self-advocacy women's group and outed ourselves publicly, we were vocal and unapologetically angry. Angry autistic women. We wanted to be heard. We were disappointed and betrayed by systems that were supposed to recognise us and help us realise our potential – as human beings, as women. Our anger was driven by the injustice done to autistic girls, teens, queer autistic people, and women. And we needed to go through that anger.

For those of you who have never experienced minority stress, I ask: *Be kind to us. Be humane. Stretch out a hand.* Offer validation and acceptance. After all we've endured, kindness can mean everything. Listen to us. Keep your hearts open. What we say isn't a personal attack – it's a plea against systemic injustice. Injustice that we, our loved ones, and autistic girls and women are still enduring.

Whenever I have the chance, I try to explain to autism professionals why we acted as we did, what it meant for our sense of self-realisation and self-acceptance, and where our minority stress came from. People who haven't faced discrimination often can't grasp the weight of minority stress or how to approach someone experiencing it.

We all need humility. We need to truly listen to one another, to keep the dialogue open, to build bridges instead of burning them.

Angela Davis, a personal inspiration of mine, said it best:

> "The way to come together is to accept difference – difference as glue, the way of coming together."

So I am not an angry autistic woman anymore.

Looking back, I see that anger was necessary. It was part of the process that all minority groups go through. But now I can reflect on which of my thoughts, actions, and words were fuelled by my own trauma. Recognising and addressing those parts of myself has been a profound step in my personal growth, one I'm deeply proud of.

I've come a long way in managing my minority stress. I've learned to stay open, to embrace new ways of thinking, and to remain flexible and fluid in my advocacy. It took psychotherapy, pharmacology, and the support of another human being – a woman, an ally, and an autism professional – who stretched out her hand and listened. She showed me how vital it is to avoid mundane us vs them divides and to instead build bridges. Together, brick by brick, we can create strong foundations. *Human connection. Difference as glue.*

This is where I am now. I'm excited to see how our minority evolves and how the bridge-building progresses.

Yet, in the face of injustice, I will still raise my voice – not out of personal anger or trauma – but from a deep empathy for those who suffer, a commitment to equity, and a belief that silence only perpetuates oppression. If, in those moments, I come across as angry or unreasonable, please ask me. Let's keep the dialogue open.

Mirror-touch synaesthesia

Mirror-touch synaesthesia is a rare form of synaesthesia where individuals experience tactile sensations on their own bodies when they observe others being touched. This phenomenon results from heightened neural activity in brain regions responsible for both observing and experiencing touch, creating a mirrored sensory response. For example, seeing someone tapped on the arm can cause a person with mirror-touch synaesthesia to feel the same sensation on their own arm. This perceptual experience reveals a strong connection between sensory processing and empathy, offering insight into how neurodivergent brains interpret sensory input.

While it can deepen interpersonal connections and enhance empathy, mirror-touch synaesthesia also presents challenges, including emotional overwhelm and social discomfort. By blurring the boundary between self and others, it provides a unique perspective on the varied ways neurodivergent individuals perceive and navigate the world.

Misgendering 🚫

Misgendering occurs when someone is referred to using incorrect gender pronouns or terms that do not align with their affirmed gender identity. It is not merely a linguistic mistake or social faux pas and can deeply affect those involved, particularly trans and non-binary individuals. Misgendering reinforces societal norms around gender conformity and can leave individuals feeling invalidated and erased.

For neurodivergent people, who may already face communication barriers and social challenges, being misgendered can amplify emotional distress and feelings of exclusion. Respecting a person's chosen name and pronouns is a fundamental act of inclusivity, affirming their identity and recognising diverse gender expressions.

Consistently using correct pronouns in daily interactions is essential for creating an environment where everyone feels acknowledged and treated with dignity.

Misophonia 💬

Misophonia is a sensory sensitivity where specific sounds trigger intense emotional reactions, such as anger, discomfort, or anxiety. It goes beyond a simple dislike of noise, stemming from neurological differences in how the brain processes auditory stimuli, particularly the connection between auditory and limbic regions.

Common triggers include everyday sounds like chewing, breathing, or tapping. These sounds can cause significant distress for neurodivergent individuals, especially those with sensory processing differences, and may disrupt daily life and relationships.

The emotional responses associated with misophonia are involuntary, driven by the nervous system's processing of sound. Recognising this highlights the need for sensory-inclusive environments that accommodate diverse auditory sensitivities.

Monotropic split 💬

A monotropic split arises within the context of monotropism, a cognitive style often seen in autistic people where the focus is intensely channelled onto a narrow range of interests or tasks. Monotropism enables a deep, immersive engagement; however, a monotropic split occurs when an individual must shift their intense focus between multiple areas of substantial interest. This can lead to strain, as the person may struggle to rapidly shift their attention, becoming mentally exhausted or overwhelmed when pushed to navigate between multiple points of focus, even when each holds significant personal value. For example, consider an autistic student who is deeply engrossed in a mathematics project and is then required to switch to an equally engaging art assignment. Even though both subjects are of high interest, the necessity to rapidly redirect focus can cause significant strain. The challenges of a monotropic split highlight the necessity of creating environments that support focused attention rather than fragment it, allowing for deeper concentration, innovative thinking, and more authentic engagement with the world.

Monotropism

Monotropism describes a narrow, intense focus of attention, commonly seen in autistic individuals. It suggests that autistic people often channel their mental resources into a limited range of interests or tasks at any given time, contrasting with the more distributed attention patterns typical of neurotypical people.

This focused attention can be both a strength and a challenge. It allows deep diving into subjects, leading to high levels of expertise and detailed understanding, often perceived as a hallmark of autistic passion and creativity. However, it can also make shifting attention to other tasks or social demands more difficult.

Understanding monotropism in autistic people enriches our appreciation of the neurodivergent mind, illustrating that what might be perceived as limitations are often just differences in cognitive processing. These insights are crucial for creating environments that respect and harness these unique cognitive profiles rather than pathologising them.

IN MY OWN WORDS: JORIS FOUET

Video games prey on me: I'm a completionist. The whole industry has optimised its addiction mechanics to a point where nothing is more important to me than getting some meaningless counter to 100%. Well, there are more important things, but it certainly doesn't seem that way.

And I found myself, time and time again, starting a game that I didn't have time to finish, and then doing nothing other than finishing it. Catastrophically failing everything else. I would spend three days barely sleeping, barely eating, just gaming until it's done. And I can't wait for it to be done. I'm not enjoying it.

But nothing trumps finishing it once I start. Which I can understand as designers doing their jobs.

But why do I start? Especially when everything else in my life is falling apart as I'm doing it.

It baffled me, but it kept happening. And at the worst times. It's like I was actively sabotaging myself.

Like I wanted the other things to fail.

And I definitely did not. Of that, I have no doubt.

I did notice that it always happened when I was spread too thin on the rest. When my attention is tugged equally by two different things, I end up stuck in the oscillation, never focusing on either. And yet, it takes all my energy to do so. I'll do anything to get out of that situation. But since neither is more important than the other, any stride in one direction is a sacrifice in the other. And I can't decide. It's not a conscious process. It's the Buridan's ass story, except it's sad because it's true.

What I can do, however, is find a third thing more important than either of those. Then at least I know what to do. At least my efforts are building to something instead of fighting against myself at every turn.

I have to finish games because the designers are pulling at my triggers. But I finally understand why I have to finish them quickly: if I don't, everything else is going to blow up. And that makes it a priority over any one of the things blowing up.

Turns out I don't play games despite their danger to me, but precisely because of it.

Prioritising is more valuable to me than achieving. They call it monotropism.

Please don't think it's a choice. I would often do anything to not struggle with that. I've lost entire careers to it.

Multigenerational trauma 🌱 🚫

This describes how trauma is passed through generations of autistic and neurodivergent people. This cycle arises when stigma, exclusion, and systemic discrimination repeatedly harm individuals, shaping not only their experiences but also the dynamics of families and communities.

For instance, an autistic person growing up in a family unaware of neurodivergence might be subjected to masking or 'behavioural corrections' to appear more neurotypical. This enforced conformity can lead to anxiety, burnout, and a loss of self. If this person becomes a parent, their unresolved trauma might affect how they engage with their autistic child – unintentionally perpetuating cycles of shame and misunderstanding.

Breaking this cycle demands systemic change: rejecting stigma, embracing neurodivergence, and creating supportive, safe and neurodivergent-affirming spaces where autistic and other neurodivergent people can live authentically and pass on acceptance rather than inherited trauma.

Multiply neurodivergent

The term 'multiply neurodivergent' describes individuals who identify with more than one form of neurodivergence, such as autism, ADHD, dyslexia, or dyspraxia. These different forms of divergence interact and influence one another, shaping each person's experiences in unique ways.

This intersection can expose individuals to compounded stigma and discrimination, as each form of neurodivergence carries distinct societal misconceptions and biases. These layers can overlap, intensifying barriers to acceptance and support. However, multiply neurodivergent individuals can also enjoy varied strengths. For example, someone who is autistic, ADHD, and dyslexic might combine the intense focus and depth of understanding often associated with autism, the rapid idea generation and spontaneous creativity linked to ADHD, and the pattern recognition and big-picture thinking commonly seen in dyslexia. This unique interplay can result in innovative problem-solving, original insights, and an ability to approach challenges from multiple, interconnected angles.

IN MY OWN WORDS: LYRIC RIVERA

I am multiply NeuroDivergent, meaning I have numerous brain differences, brain types, or NeuroTypes that shape my experiences, perspectives, and interactions with people and the world around me.

NeuroDivergent people's differences are cognitive, often invisible, and impact how we interpret and engage with the world; process information, emotions, and sensory information; and interact and communicate with others. Some NeuroDivergent people also experience neurological differences in how they experience and express movement.

Additionally, when someone is NeuroDivergent, they are often NeuroDivergent in multiple ways. Many of us have layers to our NeuroDivergence (or multiple NeuroTypes).

Many forms of NeuroDivergence are lifelong, and many people are born NeuroDivergent, but there are also types of NeuroDivergence that can be acquired through circumstances or events in life.

For me, this means living with a combination of conditions, each of which has its own unique characteristics, strengths, and challenges, and together, they create a rich tapestry that is my NeuroDivergent identity.

I am Autistic.

I am an ADHDer.

I am Hyperlexic.

I have an anxiety disorder.

I also have a "trauma brain" resulting from the mistreatment I received growing up in a world that is unkind to people who fall outside of society's norms and recurrent traumatic events that happened to me in childhood (starting before I even got to pre-school).

People who manage to grow up in circumstances where they are nurtured, experiencing minimal trauma, develop very different brains from those of us who grew up in broken homes or abusive and traumatic situations.

I was born different (Autistic) and was also pushed to diverge even further from the norm, thanks to the traumatic experiences I had during early childhood.

Being multiply NeuroDivergent means that my brain works differently from someone with only one NeuroDivergent brain type.

I perceive the world through a kaleidoscope of experiences, and my thoughts are often a whirlwind of ideas and connections (sometimes in conflict with one another).

Intense passions and interests drive me to dive deep when passionate about something.

I also have challenges with executive function, sensory processing, and emotional regulation, which can make everyday tasks and interactions feel like navigating a maze.

Autism and ADHD are both forms of NeuroDivergence I was born with (that influence my perception of the world and my communication).

I also have an anxiety disorder as well as triggers from repeated childhood trauma (that I developed from living in a world where people were cruel and unkind to me).

Whether brain differences are born or acquired throughout life, whether permanent or temporary, the more layers of NeuroDivergence a person has, the further they diverge from what is considered 'average' and the more support they will need to thrive within the systems designed by and for the NeuroTypical 'norm.'

However these brain differences originate, what matters is that each brain's owner is experiencing the world differently from those around them because no two humans (even those who share NeuroTypes) will have the exact same experience of the world.

Music therapy

Music therapy is a therapeutic practice involving the use of music to support the well-being and development of individuals. Positive outcomes are more likely when sessions align with an individual's sensory preferences and respect neurodivergent identities rather than aiming for behavioural correction or masking. Autistic individuals should feel empowered, safe, and understood in these environments. For non-speaking or minimally speaking autistic people, music therapy offers an alternative means of communication. When tied to a person's dedicated interests, it becomes even more impactful, providing a deeply personalised and meaningful experience. Applied thoughtfully, music therapy can support emotional expression, regulation, and social connection.

Myalgic encephalomyelitis

Myalgic encephalomyelitis (ME), also known as chronic fatigue syndrome (CFS), is a complex, multisystem neurological condition marked by extreme, long-lasting fatigue that does not improve with rest. This fatigue often worsens after physical or mental exertion, a phenomenon called 'post-exertional malaise.' People with ME/CFS also commonly experience sleep disturbances, muscle and joint pain, brain fog, sensitivity to light and sound, and flu-like symptoms. It can occur among individuals of any age.

The exact cause remains unclear, but ME/CFS often follows viral infections, significant physical or emotional stress, immune system dysfunction, or trauma. Genetic susceptibility may also play a role, with some research suggesting a hereditary predisposition in some individuals.

ME/CFS has no specific cure, and management focuses on symptom relief. Unfortunately, misunderstanding and stigma often surround the illness, with some healthcare providers incorrectly attributing symptoms to laziness or depression, further jeopardising patients' mental health. Concerningly, up to 90% of people with ME/CFS remain undiagnosed, making it one of the most under-recognised chronic illnesses.

National Strategy for Autistic Children, Young People, and Adults: 2021 to 2026

The National Strategy for Autistic Children, Young People, and Adults aims to improve the lives of autistic individuals in England through a structured and inclusive approach. It focuses on six key areas: enhancing public understanding and acceptance, improving educational and employment opportunities, reducing health inequalities, strengthening community support, refining systems of care, and making public spaces more inclusive for autistic people.

This strategy builds on previous initiatives, extending its scope to include children and young people for the first time rather than focusing solely on adults as earlier efforts did.

Early indications suggest some progress, particularly in raising public understanding and delivering targeted support. However, issues such as uneven service provision across regions and limited funding continue to hinder its potential. The strategy's impact will ultimately depend on effective collaboration between agencies and meaningful input from the autistic community. A full assessment of its success remains to be seen.

Nesting

Nesting refers to the instinctual act of autistic people creating a safe, organised, and highly personalised environment. It is a significant form of self-regulation, offering emotional security and comfort in a world that can often feel overwhelming due to sensory sensitivities or unexpected changes. Nesting can involve the arrangement of familiar objects, colours, or textures in a specific way that soothes the individual. The process is a natural response to the need for control over one's immediate space, helping to alleviate anxiety and enhance feelings of stability. Rather than seeing it as restrictive or obsessive, this behaviour should be respected as a legitimate expression of an autistic person's need for a predictable and calming environment.

Neuroableism 🚫

Neuroableism refers to the prejudice and discrimination faced by neurodivergent individuals, particularly autistic people, due to societal preferences for neurotypical traits and behaviours. It stems from the belief that neurotypical ways of thinking, communicating, and interacting are superior to those of neurodivergent people. This bias can manifest in various ways, from everyday interactions to institutional policies (resulting in 'structural neuroableism'), often marginalising neurodivergent individuals and pressuring them to 'fit in' with neurotypical norms. Neuroableism often drives attempts to 'normalise' neurodivergent people through therapies aimed at masking their natural traits, which can be damaging to the self-esteem and mental health of neurodivergent people.

Neuroclearing 🧠

Neuroclearing is a concept that describes the natural need for certain neurodivergent individuals, especially autistic people, to engage in activities that help clear internal 'neurological traffic.' These activities might include stimming, verbal echolalia, or engaging in routines or interests. Such behaviours serve a crucial self-regulatory function, enabling the brain to process and release accumulated sensory, emotional, or cognitive stimuli. Without this neuroclearing, neurological pathways can become overloaded, leading to heightened stress, anxiety, and an increased likelihood of meltdowns or shutdowns. Recognising this process as essential for maintaining neurological balance highlights the importance of accepting and supporting these behaviours as part of an individual's natural coping mechanisms rather than viewing them as something to suppress.

Neurocosmopolitanism ⚖️

Neurocosmopolitanism refers to the idea of embracing and valuing neurodiversity on a global scale. The concept promotes an inclusive mindset that recognises the full spectrum of neurological differences, such as autism, ADHD, and dyslexia, as natural variations of human brains rather than deficits or conditions to be 'fixed.' The term calls for the cultivation of a world where neurodivergent people can coexist with neurotypical individuals in a spirit of mutual respect and understanding, without the stigma or forced conformity that often accompanies these differences.

Neurodivergent and neurodivergence 🧠

The terms 'neurodivergent' and 'neurodivergence' describe differences in neurological development and identity compared to what is considered typical or 'neurotypical.' 'Neurodivergent' refers to individuals whose neurological experiences differ from neurotypical individuals, such as autistic, ADHD, dyslexic, and Tourette's individuals. Neurodivergence, on the other hand, refers to the broader concept of these differences, encompassing both the diversity of neurological states and the experiences shaped by them.

These concepts challenge traditional ideas of neurological 'normalcy.' They emphasise that many difficulties arise not from an individual's neurology itself but from a mismatch between their neurological needs and societal expectations, environments, and values.

Neurodivergence is not a monolith. Each individual's reality is shaped by the interplay of their specific neurotype, personality, socio-cultural context, and other identity factors, resulting in highly varied and deeply personal experiences.

IN MY OWN WORDS: GINNY GRANT

Let's start with a short lesson in history. The term 'neurodivergent' was coined by American Autism rights activist Kassiane Asasumasu (formerly Kassiane Sibley) around the year 2000. Asasumasu recognised that many people are 'neurologically divergent from typical,' not just Autistic people. Asasumasu stated that 'neurodivergent' was a term that could be applied to all kinds of individuals whose brains differed from the dominant neurotype: Autistic people; ADHDers; those with learning disabilities, epilepsy, dyspraxia, mental illness, MS, Parkinson's and more. Importantly, Asasumasu argued, neurodivergence is a tool of inclusion, not one of exclusion. Asasumasu's work led to a more encompassing understanding and acceptance of neurological differences and gave activists a way to advocate for rights and accommodations for all of those people whose neurocognitive functioning differs from the norm.

In addition to crediting Kassiane Asasumasu, I'd like to also acknowledge the more recent work of neurodivergent advocate and author, Sonny Jane Wise (@livedexperienceeducator), who has tirelessly argued for a broader conception of the terms 'neurodivergent' and 'neurodivergence.'

Initially after my Autism diagnosis, I identified simply as Autistic. But in the five years that have followed my diagnosis, things have shifted for me, and I now refer to myself more commonly as 'neurodivergent,' because I know my brain diverges in multiple complex ways from the dominant neurotypical majority. In addition to Autism, I have received diagnoses of major depressive disorder (MDD), EDNOS, OCD and PTSD – and I specifically include my mental health diagnoses, because I know that these, too, impact greatly how I think, feel, communicate, and socialise. Furthermore, I know that having a neurodivergent brain doesn't mean there is anything wrong with me as such, although I accept there are times when it can be difficult. As Sonny Jane Wise says in their recent title *We're All Neurodiverse*: "Identifying as neurodivergent means being able to understand, address and accept the challenges you might've faced in life without having to view yourself as the problem. It's a lens through which you can understand your differences and needs, and that you move through this world and function differently."

Neurodivergent-affirming ⚖️ 🛡️

The term 'neurodivergent-affirming' refers to practices, policies, and approaches that validate, support, and celebrate neurodivergence. This perspective emphasises the inherent value and strengths of individuals with neurodivergent identities. Instead of viewing these identities as deficits or disorders that need to be corrected, these approaches recognise, accommodate and leverage the unique ways of thinking, learning, and interacting with the world. In education, this might include flexible seating, assistive technology, and teacher training on neurodiversity. Identity-first language, inclusive environments, and an understanding of neuroableism are central principles. By embracing neurodivergence, neurodivergent-affirming approaches aim to dismantle stigma, empower individuals, and ensure respect and understanding for all neurodivergent people.

IN MY OWN WORDS: ADITI GANGRADE

When I first encountered the term 'neurodivergent-affirming' and grasped its meaning, my initial thought was, "Isn't this just common courtesy?"

To my surprise, it wasn't. My partner Aalap often says, "The things that come naturally to us, like being neurodivergent-affirming, are seen as 'extra efforts' or 'DEI initiatives' for many non-neurodivergent people."

Realizing that most spaces and systems are far from affirming, we decided to champion this cause through our company Much Much Media.

Film sets, for example, are often a sensory overload – too chaotic to ask for clear, repeated instructions or to take breaks when needed. Yelling is common, and if you dare ask for accommodations, you're told, "Why work in the media industry if you have communication difficulties?"

People often fail to realize that small adjustments – whether it's written instructions or sensory breaks – can enable neurodivergent creatives to excel. Sometimes, they'll outperform expectations when given the right support.

At Much Much Spectrum, we've committed to making all our spaces – work environments, sets, meetings – neurodivergent-friendly. Our crews are sensitized to ensure these spaces are judgment-free, affirming, and adaptable to each person's individual needs. Even our content aims to dismantle biases that feed into neuronormativity. We start by embracing those who don't fit societal molds, who have marginalized identities, and creating room for them to thrive.

One vivid memory from my childhood stays with me.

I often came home from school in tears for different reasons, but one day was particularly bad. My mom sat with me as we had lunch, trying to understand what had upset me. That day, I couldn't stop crying. I told her that when teachers spoke, I often didn't catch their words the first time. When I asked my math teacher to repeat something, she snapped at me in front of the class. I was humiliated. And it wasn't just that moment – there were many things about me that others seemed to find 'weird.'

"Why am I the only one with all these problems?" I asked my mom. She replied, "These aren't problems; they're just your needs." She spoke to my teacher, but more than that, my parents always focused on my strengths. They raised me with a sense of respect and confidence, especially in front of others. Even when I got scolded at home, they never demeaned me in public. I didn't see that level of support from many other parents around me.

That experience changed everything. My parents' unwavering belief in me helped me rise from my darkest moments. Today, I carry that same neurodivergent-affirming attitude into all my relationships – with my partner, family, team, and friends.

I approach everyone with curiosity, seeking to understand rather than judge, free of neuronormative expectations.

Neurodiversity

Neurodiversity is a concept that recognises the natural variation in human brains and neurological systems and challenges the idea that there is an inherently 'right' or 'normal' way for these systems to function. It asserts that neurological differences, including autism, ADHD, dyslexia, and others, are simply part of the spectrum of human diversity and identity. Rather than viewing neurodivergent people as deficient or disordered, neurodiversity promotes acceptance of these differences, much like biodiversity is valued in nature.

The concept of neurodiversity rejects the medical model of disability, which focuses on 'fixing,' 'treating,' or 'curing' those who deviate from neurotypical norms. Instead, it emphasises the need for societal change to support and celebrate all types of neurological configurations. In this way, neurodiversity calls for a shift in thinking – promoting equality, equity, dignity, and full inclusion for all individuals including those who are neurodivergent.

Neurodiversity-aware curriculum design

Neurodiversity-aware curriculum design creates educational programmes that recognise and value neurological differences as natural aspects of human diversity. It is grounded in the neurodiversity paradigm, which views variations in how people process information – such as those seen in autistic and other neurodivergent people – as natural and valuable aspects of human diversity.

This approach adapts to individual learning styles, sensory needs, and communication preferences rather than aiming to 'normalise' students. By removing barriers that cause marginalisation, it enables an inclusive and respectful learning environment. Key elements might include flexible instructional methods, the use of assistive technologies, and the creation of spaces where sensory sensitivities are acknowledged, supported, and, as much as possible, leveraged.

Neurofibromatosis

Neurofibromatosis is a group of genetic conditions primarily impacting the growth and development of nerve cells, leading to the formation of benign tumours on nerves throughout the body. Symptoms range from skin changes to neurological complications. The two main types, NF1 and NF2, each with varying degrees of impact, can lead to hearing loss, vision problems, and learning differences. NF1, the most common form, may also impact bone development, cardiovascular health, and cognitive health. Women with NF1 face a higher risk of breast cancer, particularly between ages 30 and 40. While lifelong, its effects vary widely, from minimal symptoms to requiring significant medical intervention. Despite affecting over 2 million people globally, awareness remains low.

Neurofuturism ⚖️

Neurofuturism is concept that intersects with both the neurodiversity paradigm and future technological advancements. It envisions a world where neurodivergent people, such as autistic individuals, are not only accepted but actively involved in shaping the future through their unique cognitive perspectives. This idea highlights the potential of neurodivergent thought patterns, which often challenge traditional ways of problem-solving and innovation, as assets in navigating and transforming future societal and technological landscapes.

Neuroharmony ⚖️

The concept of neuroharmony refers to an ideal state where all neurotypes are embraced and integrated into society without judgement or discrimination. It promotes the value of all neurological differences, recognising that the coexistence of diverse ways of thinking can create a richer, more inclusive community. In a neuroharmonious society, environments are designed to support and celebrate diverse needs rather than forcing conformity to a neurotypical standard.

Neurokin 👥

The term 'neurokin' refers to individuals who share a bond through their mutual neurodivergent identities, recognising their shared experiences of navigating a world predominantly shaped by neurotypical norms. Being neurokin transcends specific diagnoses; it speaks to a kinship among those who understand what it means to think, feel, and process the world differently. The term, therefore, embraces a sense of community and solidarity, recognising that neurodivergent people, including autistic individuals, benefit from connections with others who experience similar societal challenges.

Neurokin magnetism 👥

Neurokin magnetism refers to the natural tendency of neurodivergent people to gravitate towards one another, often without conscious awareness of their shared neurodivergence. Autistic and ADHD individuals, for example, may unknowingly form friendships, relationships, or communities that ease communication barriers linked to the double empathy problem.

This attraction, or magnetism, could serve as a neurological defence mechanism, allowing neurodivergent individuals to experience greater understanding and acceptance from those with similar cognitive processes. In today's interconnected world, particularly through social media, these dynamics are more visible and available than ever before. The increase in neurodivergent connections may also contribute to the rise in neurodivergent identities and diagnoses, as more neurodivergent parents find each other, leading to more neurodivergent children. However, the primary driver behind this rise remains society's improved understanding of neurodivergence.

Neurology

Neurology refers to the study and understanding of the brain, nervous system, and the complex network of nerves that shape human behaviour, thought processes, and sensory interactions. Traditionally, neurology has been dedicated to identifying and treating conditions like epilepsy, multiple sclerosis, and stroke, often viewing neurological variations primarily as deviations from a 'normal' standard. However, this pathological focus has inadvertently overlooked the strengths and intrinsic value of diverse neurological configurations, thereby contributing to the medicalisation of neurodivergent identities, such as autism and ADHD.

Neuronormativity

The term 'neuronormativity' refers to the societal belief that neurotypical ways of thinking, behaving, and processing information are the ideal standard. This assumption positions neurotypical people as the default and frames neurological differences, such as autism, as deviations that need to be corrected. The concept upholds neuroableism by perpetuating the idea that neurotypical traits are superior and should be the standard, sidelining and disadvantaging neurodivergent individuals. Challenging this perspective is essential to creating a more inclusive view of human diversity – one that recognises all forms of neurological functioning, whether neurotypical or neurodivergent, as equally valuable.

Neurophobia

Neurophobia describes a fear or discomfort towards neurological concepts, including neurodivergent identities like autism. This reluctance to engage with or learn about neurodiversity often reinforces misconceptions and stigma, especially in educational, medical, and professional settings. The prevalence of neurophobia is particularly high among medical students and doctors, likely because understanding neurological differences requires unlearning ingrained medical-model perspectives and adopting a more critical, inclusive approach. Effective training depends on educators who embrace neurodivergence rather than those who reinforce deficit-focused frameworks, which remain dominant in medical education.

Neuroplasticity

Neuroplasticity refers to the brain's ability to reorganise and form new connections in response to experiences, learning, and changes in the environment. It highlights the adaptability of neural pathways, meaning the brain is not a static organ but is continuously evolving throughout a person's life. This process is crucial for learning new skills, recovery after brain injuries, and the brain's response to sensory or cognitive challenges. Neuroplasticity can also be seen as a mechanism that supports diverse ways of processing and interacting with the world.

Neuroqueering and neuroqueerness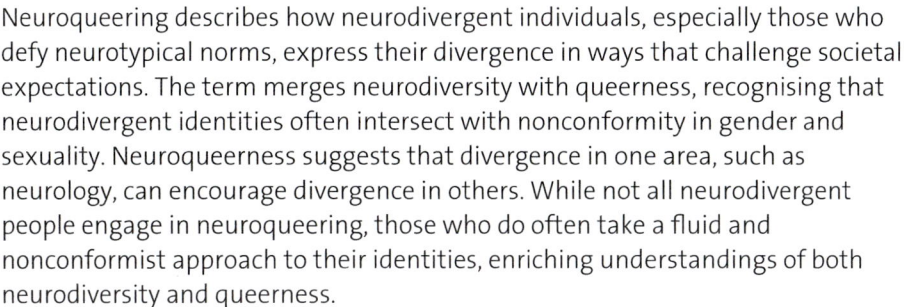

Neuroqueering describes how neurodivergent individuals, especially those who defy neurotypical norms, express their divergence in ways that challenge societal expectations. The term merges neurodiversity with queerness, recognising that neurodivergent identities often intersect with nonconformity in gender and sexuality. Neuroqueerness suggests that divergence in one area, such as neurology, can encourage divergence in others. While not all neurodivergent people engage in neuroqueering, those who do often take a fluid and nonconformist approach to their identities, enriching understandings of both neurodiversity and queerness.

An autistic person who openly hand flaps in public, reclaiming this joyful and self-regulating behaviour despite societal pressure to suppress it, demonstrates neuroqueering. Similarly, a neurodivergent therapist who integrates their unique cognitive style into their practice challenges conventional norms within mental health. Both examples illustrate how neuroqueering reclaims authenticity while reshaping societal expectations.

IN MY OWN WORDS: ADITI GANGRADE

In school, there were always these unspoken norms everyone just seemed to know instinctively.

I, however, struggled to catch on. Changing schools nine times during my school years didn't help. Each one had its own set of unwritten rules, and I couldn't keep up.

But one thing was constant: neuronormativity and heteronormativity. No one could even imagine a high school girl having a crush on another girl. When someone talked about crushes, it was always, "Who's the boy?" as if anything else was unthinkable.

Same-sex relationships didn't even cross our minds.

I was a high-masking girl, meaning my neurodivergence and queerness were invisible to others because I worked hard every day to fit in.

In high school, there was a girl in my class who had an intellectual disability. She looked different, had darker skin, and came from a marginalized caste. Back then, I didn't fully understand the significance of her multiple identities.

She was always alone – during assembly, recess, just . . . by herself. No one spoke to her, and she had no friends. I never approached her either because I was afraid that if I did, I'd be excluded from the tiny circle of people I called 'friends' back then.

That was also the time puberty hit. Suddenly, I had to deal with menstruation and body changes. It was awful. I hated wearing pads – periods were a sensory nightmare for me. And then came the bra. I remember flat-out refusing to wear one. I had a meltdown almost every day for a month. I already disliked school, and this made it so much worse.

No one understood my sensory sensitivities. That's when my anger started to show. All the emotions I had been masking for years began to spill out in the form of outbursts.

I often heard things like, "Anger doesn't suit girls," or "No one will marry you if you keep throwing tantrums," from my aunts. I was only 13! Who says that to a kid?

While I was battling the tight, uncomfortable bra, annoyed all the time, snapping at everyone around me, the girl from my batch – the one I mentioned earlier – wasn't doing any of that. She didn't follow the rules. She didn't wear what was expected of her, didn't mask her differences. And she seemed happy, sitting alone, eating alone, going home alone.

Growing up in convent schools, rules, norms, and restrictions were drilled into me. I began to believe that adulthood would be the same – no freedom to be different, no space for anything outside of the cis-het norm. It was suffocating.

But after I graduated, I started to see that the world isn't just black and white. I realized I could embrace the gray areas, that I could be different.

Now, at 26, as a neuroqueer entrepreneur and filmmaker, I've made it my mission to break these normative molds – one story at a time.

Neurospicy

'Neurospicy' is an informal term used to describe neurodivergent experiences, often in a playful or self-affirming way. It emerged in online spaces as an alternative to clinical or stigmatising labels and can offer a lighthearted means of self-expression while avoiding specific diagnostic disclosure. However, the term has drawn criticism for framing neurodivergence as something quirky or amusing, which can trivialise the serious challenges many neurodivergent people face. This framing often contributes to infantilisation, reducing neurodivergent adults to childlike or unserious figures, particularly those with higher support needs or those who cannot live independently. For many, more established terms like 'neurodivergent' are preferred for their clarity, inclusivity, and resistance to euphemism.

Neurotypical

The term 'neurotypical' refers to individuals whose neurological development and processes align with what is generally considered the societal majority and thus norm. This concept contrasts to 'neurodivergent' which describes those whose neurology processes differently. Neurotypical individuals may experience fewer barriers in navigating social life because environments and society are designed with their needs prioritised, which can lead to societal structures that disable neurodivergent people.

Nociceptive sense

The nociceptive sense refers to the sensory system responsible for detecting and processing stimuli related to pain, injury, or potential harm. It alerts the brain to harmful physical stimuli, enabling the body to respond and protect itself. Unlike other senses that primarily deal with external perceptions (such as sight or sound), nociception is a critical internal mechanism for signalling damage, either from external factors like heat or internal issues such as inflammation.

Autistic individuals often experience non-typical nociception, with some showing heightened pain sensitivity (hypersensitivity) and others reduced sensitivity (hyposensitivity). These differences can result in responses to pain or injury that defy typical expectations. Additionally, many autistic individuals experience alexithymia, which is a difficulty in identifying or describing their emotions, including the sensation of pain. This can further complicate how pain is communicated and understood, potentially leading to misunderstandings in healthcare or support settings.

Nomatnesia

Nomatnesia refers to the specific challenge of recalling names, derived from the Latin 'nomen' (name) and 'amnesia' (forgetfulness). Autistic people and other neurodivergent individuals may experience nomatnesia due to differences in processing and retaining verbal or social information. This can sometimes lead to social misunderstandings or embarrassment, particularly in cultures where remembering names is highly valued. Strategies such as associating names with visual cues or keeping written notes can mitigate these challenges. Looking ahead, assistive technologies like augmented reality glasses could play a role in providing real-time reminders of people's names during conversations, offering practical solutions for those who experience nomatnesia.

Non-speaking people

The term 'non-speaking' people describes individuals who do not use verbal speech as their primary method of communication. This does not indicate a lack of intelligence or cognitive ability; non-speaking people are often just as articulate, thoughtful, and capable of complex reasoning as those who speak verbally.

Non-speaking autistic individuals frequently communicate through augmentative and alternative communication (AAC), sign language, written text, or other non-verbal tools. These methods are valid, meaningful, and effective, allowing individuals to express their thoughts, preferences, and emotions clearly.

However, societal emphasis on spoken communication creates significant barriers. Non-speaking communication is often misunderstood, undervalued, and met with stigma. These attitudes result in reduced support, respect, and inclusion for non-speaking individuals, making societal attitudes the primary disabling factor rather than the non-speaking identity itself.

Non-speaking people have internal voices, opinions, and preferences. While some may also have learning disabilities, this is equally true for speaking individuals. Misconceptions persist, often assuming intellectual disability where none exists, reinforcing harmful stereotypes.

The term 'non-speaking' has replaced 'non-verbal' to better reflect lived experiences. Non-verbal suggests an absence of communication or verbal comprehension, which is inaccurate for many non-speaking people. They may have strong verbal comprehension and express themselves effectively using AAC or typing. The term 'non-speaking' avoids ableist assumptions, highlights the richness of diverse communication styles, and promotes a more accurate and respectful understanding.

IN MY OWN WORDS: BEN BREAUX

When I was young, around 1.5–2 years old, I had rather full – even advanced – out loud speech. I would say analogies, sing songs, and go up to people on the street to strike up a conversation. Because of this, I am quite aware of what it means to be considered a speaking member of society. However, when I was about 2.5 years old, what is known as "Regressive Autism" kicked in. While it is still up for debate why this happens, it meant a severe reduction in communication and perceived social skills. I then discovered this meant a severe decline in educational opportunities. Suddenly it was deemed by society that I no longer had the capacity for – or interest in – learning, which is quite far from the truth.

Having this label now meant that those in the Public School System mostly looked at my 'Deficiencies and Behaviors' instead of my Intelligence and Considerable Abilities. Because I was predominantly identified as a 'Non-verbal' Student (and please note it should always be the use of the phrase 'NonSPEAKING' as I know how to use words, I just can't SPEAK them) it was determined I would only be able to have access to a 'Life Skills'–based curriculum. I know Life Skills should be an important part of any young person's education, and I greatly appreciated learning how to do some of them, yet, much more actual ACADEMIC CONTENT should also be available and accessible to students like me.

Once I was fluent in using the Letter Board to communicate, my Mom arranged for one of my Communication/Regulation Partners to do a demonstration with me of a complex academic lesson in front of teachers and staff at the school. The lesson incorporated the use and knowledge of high-level Math and Language Skills. All present were in agreement that I, myself, was actually doing the academic work presented and granted me 10 minutes (yes ONLY 10!) of 'academics' a day, when possible. These lessons consisted of my teacher reading me a piece about a topic (often that my Mom had sent in) and then me answering a few multiple choice questions correctly. Even though these lessons were short, I so adored and valued them! They were so much better than spending hours sitting at a table stuffing envelopes with blank pieces of folded paper or doing other well intended but very mundane 'busy work' tasks. Sadly, while I treasured it so, this 'Academic Allowance' was only given for one year and then replaced with me independently watching videos on YouTube 'to increase my Leisure Skills' (which was what my academic lessons were formally under in my IEP!). The school told us, "When it comes down to it, for the kids like Ben in the Autism Program, we are a Life Skills–based program because research shows this is the best way for them to succeed."

My IQ tests were wrongfully and unfairly given by demanding spoken out loud responses. Consequently, my scores appeared as very low thus giving further 'proof' to society and the education system that I was not worthy of an academic education.

I decided that they were wrong and was determined to fight to get a proper education suitable for someone with my capabilities. To be blatantly honest, sometimes it was a nightmare. The public school system belittled me into thinking I amounted to nothing.

With the strong support of an 'in the educational system' ally, I convinced my County Public School System to allow me to take the statewide assessments with a trained CRP and FULL ACCESS to all the necessary Letter Boards (composition, math, etc). I came out at 82% in comparison to all 18-year-old United States Public School Students! Even after knowing my test results, I was told I would still have to take 'Adaptive' courses and would not have access to General Studies. So, I found a program that allows me to get my full academic based high school diploma. It is virtual and has self-paced components. Now that I am being given the proper academic resources and supports, I have finally been able to prove my educational abilities and to truly succeed in learning and attending a school program, which is so much more than what would've come from staying in public school. To me, it seems very sad that I had to do so very much self-advocacy to have access to a real education. I hope the future holds a reverence and respect for PRESUME COMPETENCE and that others like me are giving better and much more equitable educational opportunities as I – and all others – so deserve.

As human beings, we non, minimally, and unreliably speaking autistics have the right to equally multifaceted, and fulfilling lives, and – with accommodations, appropriate supports, and true faith in and understanding of our abilities – this is entirely possible!

I want to take a moment to share a quote from something my Mom wrote that resonates for me, *"If, as a society, we continue to see the limits of Autistics – particularly by attributing labels of 'Intellectual Disability' or 'Low Functioning,' and fail to see the incredible brilliance within . . . we are just perpetuating a crime of double damage; with both the Autistics – and all of us, potentially losing out on truly knowing what are incredible, concerned, giving, intelligent minds with the hearts, souls and brains to contribute greatly to the world around us all. Stop negating. Start engaging and seeking now."*

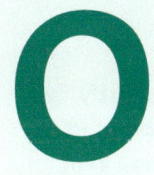

Obsessions

The term 'obsessions' is often misused to describe the intense focus many autistic people have on specific topics or activities. This focus is not pathological but frequently a source of joy, learning, and expertise. What others label as obsessions are often better understood as expressions of monotropism – a cognitive tendency to concentrate deeply on fewer interests at a time.

Such concentration enables rich, immersive experiences and often results in exceptional skill or knowledge in areas of passion. Framing these interests negatively reinforces misconceptions, suggesting they are maladaptive or require intervention. In reality, they should be recognised and valued for their contributions to both individual fulfilment and societal innovation.

Obsessive compulsive disorder

Obsessive compulsive disorder (OCD) is a form of neurodivergence characterised by persistent, intrusive thoughts and compulsive behaviours that individuals feel driven to perform. Increasingly recognised within the neurodiversity framework, OCD is understood as a reflection of neurological uniqueness rather than merely a disorder. Compulsions often serve as coping mechanisms for deep-rooted anxiety, trauma, or distress, offering a sense of control in environments where control feels absent or suppressed.

For many autistic and neurodivergent people, these compulsions are linked to experiences of stigma and marginalisation. Day-to-day activities and overall well-being can be significantly affected. Popular culture frequently misrepresents OCD as an exaggerated preference for cleanliness or order, trivialising its complexity. A more accurate understanding requires empathy, meaningful support, and resources that empower individuals to manage OCD and lead fulfilling lives on their own terms.

IN MY OWN WORDS: GINNY GRANT

I discovered I have obsessive compulsive disorder at the age of 39, shortly before I was identified as Autistic. My OCD diagnosis was a pivotal point in my life: it explained decades of obsessions and compulsions that I had kept secret, as I knew they weren't thoughts or acts that the average person experienced, but I didn't quite know what they signified.

One aspect of my OCD is disturbing images of knives and blood. These can come at any moment in my day, often while performing a task as benign and mundane as taking a shower or doing the dishes. I am quick to suppress these intrusive thoughts. Another aspect of my OCD is repeated lock checking. This, I have done daily from the age of about 10, and I will not go to sleep unless I am satisfied that I have thoroughly (repeatedly) checked all the possible entry points in my location. It was only when the compulsions really took over – in the form of rigorously tracking my food and exercising – that I came to see these various 'secret' aspects of my experience for what they were, that is, characteristic of OCD. Forget the stereotype of obsessive cleaning: these particular compulsions had dangerous consequences for my health.

With the support of my psychiatrist, GP, and psychologist, I have learned that a combination of psychotropic medications and psychotherapy are what is needed to keep my OCD under control. Occasionally my internalised ableism pops up to tell me that I should not need this kind of medication, but I try to remind myself that I function better, I live better, when the OCD is well-managed and medication plays an important role in that.

One aspect of having OCD that I have had to accept is its impact on my ability to focus. My psychiatrist refers to 'OCD chatter in the brain,' and I know exactly what this 'chatter' is like. It can be very hard to concentrate when your brain is processing all this other stuff while trying to go about your daily life. So I have learned to be gentle with myself and not judgemental when I am struggling to focus with all the 'chatter' going on in my brain.

Occupational therapy

Occupational therapy (OT) involves a wide range of strategies designed to support people in improving their ability to engage in everyday activities. While often associated with skills like dressing, writing, and task organisation, its role within the neurodivergent community is broader. For autistic people, OT may address sensory integration, communication, and environmental adaptations to reduce sensory overload or anxiety.

Occupational therapists collaborate with individuals to identify barriers and develop personalised solutions that enhance autonomy and comfort. Neurodivergent-affirming OT avoids attempts to normalise behaviour, instead focusing on respecting individual needs, enabling self-regulation, and empowering people to live authentically.

Olfactory sense

The olfactory sense refers to the ability to perceive smells and plays a significant role in sensory processing. For autistic people, olfactory sensitivity can vary greatly, with some experiencing heightened reactions to smells that others might find mild or neutral, sometimes leading to sensory overload. Others may have reduced sensitivity and seek out strong scents for sensory input.

Smell is deeply linked to memory and emotion, as the olfactory bulb connects closely with the hippocampus and amygdala – areas of the brain responsible for these functions. This connection can make certain smells evoke intense emotional responses or vivid memories, which may be particularly pronounced in neurodivergent individuals.

Oliver McGowan training ⚖️ 🏢

The Oliver McGowan Mandatory Training is a UK initiative designed to improve understanding of neurodivergent people, particularly autistic individuals and those with learning disabilities, within health and social care. Named after Oliver McGowan, an autistic teenager with a learning disability who died in 2016 due to inadequate care, the training aims to prevent similar failures.

Paula McGowan, Oliver's mother, played a central role in campaigning for this change, leading to its statutory inclusion in the Health and Care Act 2022. The Act mandates all regulated health and social care providers to ensure their staff receive appropriate training, with the Oliver McGowan Mandatory Training serving as the UK government's preferred programme to meet this requirement.

Co-designed with autistic people and those with learning disabilities, the training integrates their lived experiences to ensure accurate and empathetic representation. It is delivered in two tiers, both beginning with an e-learning module. Tier 1 includes a one-hour online interactive session, co-delivered by an autistic person and/or a person with a learning disability alongside a facilitator. Tier 2 involves a one-day face-to-face session, also co-delivered by an autistic person and/or a person with a learning disability alongside a trainer. This structure ensures authenticity is embedded throughout the programme.

Implementation is coordinated through integrated care boards, with a focus on building capacity by training trainers, including those with lived experience. This co-production approach goes beyond symbolism, equipping healthcare workers with practical skills and a deeper understanding to bridge the gap between them and the neurodivergent community.

Online learning

Online learning refers to the delivery of education through digital platforms, allowing learners and instructors to engage remotely rather than in traditional classroom settings. It often forms part of hybrid models that combine online sessions with face-to-face teaching. For neurodivergent learners, including autistic people, online learning offers flexibility, self-paced access to materials, and tools tailored to sensory and cognitive needs. This creates a more accessible learning environment where content can be revisited and engagement happens on individual terms. However, challenges around communication and interaction remain, as online spaces can lack the personal connection or sensory considerations some learners require. Success depends on thoughtful design that accommodates diverse learning styles, ensuring everyone feels supported and able to participate fully.

Onychophagia

Onychophagia, commonly referred to as nail-biting, is a compulsive behaviour characterised by the chronic biting of one's nails. Many neurodivergent individuals use it as a form of stimming, particularly those with heightened oral or tactile sensitivities. For them, nail-biting is not just a habit but a way to manage sensory overload or emotional discomfort, offering brief relief in overwhelming moments.

Supporting someone with onychophagia often means adjusting their environment and offering alternative sensory tools, like tactile toys, rather than trying to eliminate the behaviour entirely. Viewing it as a valid coping strategy rather than a problem to fix, encourages a more inclusive and compassionate approach.

IN MY OWN WORDS: JORIS FOUET

I've always bitten my nails. But I stopped hurting myself with it when I was 11. It had been a whole ordeal. I had, for a few years, on a regular basis, been drawing blood from trimming my nails. I would literally have wounds that took days to heal from me taking bites out of myself.

It did not make much sense. But it was there.

Basically, I would trim my nails properly. And then I would start again. Except there was nothing left to remove, but I really wanted to. So I took away too much.

I think there were two forces at play: the need for stim and the need for control.

I'm a stimmer: I am drawn to specific sensory perceptions. The feeling of it happening is soothing to me. And I needed a lot of soothing as a kid. Somehow the feeling of tearing keratin falls in that category.

I'm also a control freak. There were a lot of things I did not understand about maintaining my body, but making sure I didn't have nails too long was one of the few things I had a hand in. So I overdid it. I checked because it was good to check. And I rechecked after checking, and "better safe than sorry" told me I should go too far just in case.

After years of trying everything we could to overcome this as a family, at 11 I just realised that it was, in fact, detrimental in the long run, regardless of how it seemed in the short run. And I stopped overdoing it overnight. I still have the same draw to it. I just stopped trusting that craving.

Nowadays, it's a managed addiction. I still do it, but I don't hurt myself. It's a little ceremony. I prepare it, make sure the time is right, that nothing will disturb me. I enjoy it thoroughly. I'm just very clear that when it's done, it's done. And any further temptation is stifled by merely looking forward to the next session.

Still, to this day, you couldn't make me use a nail trimmer to save my life.

Outness 👥 ⚖️ 💧

In neurodiversity contexts, outness refers to how openly someone shares their neurodivergent identity. It is tied to living authentically without masking traits to meet neurotypical expectations. For many autistic people, being 'out' is an act of self-acceptance and a rejection of societal pressures to camouflage their differences.

Outness can strengthen connections within the autistic community, reduce isolation, and contribute to normalising neurodivergent identities. However, it is a deeply personal choice, influenced by context, safety, and the attitudes of those around them.

Overstimulation and understimulation 🧠 🌿

Overstimulation and understimulation describe how neurodivergent individuals experience sensory input. Overstimulation occurs when sensory input – like light, sound, or touch – becomes overwhelming, often leading to stress, anxiety, or shutdowns as the brain struggles to process excessive stimuli. Understimulation, in contrast, happens when sensory input is insufficient, causing discomfort or frustration.

Sensory experiences can also accumulate over time, a phenomenon referred to as 'accumulated stimulation,' which may result in overwhelm if not addressed. These differences stem from heightened or diminished sensory sensitivities, shaping how autistic individuals engage with their surroundings.

Because sensory needs vary between individuals, effective strategies often require flexibility. Holistic approaches, such as mindfulness, exercise, and nature therapy, can help manage sensory challenges. Creating environments that respect and accommodate these needs is essential for promoting safety, comfort, and overall well-being.

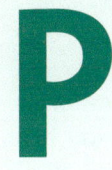

P

Panic attack 🌿 🚫

A panic attack is a sudden and intense surge of fear or discomfort, usually peaking within minutes. Common symptoms include a rapid heart rate, sweating, trembling, teeth chattering, and shortness of breath. While often linked to anxiety, neurodivergent individuals, particularly autistic people, may experience panic attacks due to sensory overload, executive function demands, or overwhelming environments.

The body's fight-or-flight response activates during these episodes, even without an immediate threat. Autistic individuals are often more vulnerable due to anxiety linked to changes in routine, communication difficulties, or sensory sensitivities, making unpredictable or chaotic situations more likely triggers.

People with somatic alexithymia – difficulty recognising and describing physical sensations, especially those related to illness or discomfort – may not realise they are experiencing a panic attack. This can delay self-soothing or seeking help, adding to the distress.

Immediate support focuses on creating calm, predictable environments and offering grounding techniques such as controlled breathing or sensory anchors. Safe redirection of thoughts by a trusted person can also help, providing gentle reassurance or guiding focus away from overwhelming sensations. Providing options for sensory regulation – such as noise-cancelling headphones, weighted items, or a quieter space – can further reduce anxiety.

Long-term strategies may include evaluating environmental and systemic factors to prevent recurring triggers. Patience, compassion, and a non-judgemental approach remain essential, as pressure or negative reactions can intensify distress.

Parallel play and interactive play 👥

Parallel play and interactive play describe different ways children engage with others. In parallel play, children play side by side without directly interacting. They might use the same space and similar toys but remain focused on their own activity. This is typical in early childhood and reflects a different way of engaging with the environment, not a lack of social interest.

Interactive play, on the other hand, involves direct communication, cooperation, and shared activities. It requires a wider range of social interaction skills and mutual involvement. Both forms of play can be meaningful for autistic children, and transitioning between them may take time depending on their sensory and social needs. It is important to respect these differences and avoid pressuring children into a style of play they are not ready for.

Parent and family advocacy

Parent and family advocacy is a key aspect of the broader neurodiversity movement, where parents, carers, and families actively support the rights and inclusion of their autistic family members. This type of advocacy involves publicly championing the acceptance of autistic people, raising awareness of their unique strengths and challenges, and fighting against stigma and discrimination. Family advocates often work to ensure that systems like education, healthcare, and employment become more accessible and supportive for autistic individuals. Importantly, parent and family advocacy must centre the voices and perspectives of autistic people themselves.

Parkinson's

Parkinson's is a neurological phenomenon primarily associated with movement and motor control. It involves the gradual degeneration of nerve cells in a specific area of the brain, leading to symptoms like tremors, stiffness, and difficulty with balance and coordination. Parkinson's, however, is not just about motor issues; it can also affect mood, cognition, and sensory experiences.

Autistic people are three times more likely to develop Parkinson's-like symptoms ('parkinsonism') than non-autistics. This highlights the importance of careful neurological assessment for autistic people, particularly as they age, to distinguish between autism-related motor differences and neurodegenerative conditions like Parkinson's. While Parkinson's presents significant challenges, each person's experience is unique and should not be reduced to the condition alone.

Peer advocacy

Peer advocacy involves autistic or neurodivergent individuals supporting each other to navigate challenges, assert their rights, and have their voices heard. Unlike traditional advocacy, peer advocates share lived experiences with those they support, creating a deeper understanding and connection. This relationship can empower individuals to articulate their needs and access resources while validating their unique perspectives. Equality underpins peer advocacy and enables spaces where neurodivergent people can be authentic without fear of judgement or imposed expectations. Peer advocacy occurs in settings like education, workplaces, and healthcare, playing a crucial role in reducing stigma and encouraging acceptance.

Peer education

Peer education is a collaborative learning process where individuals within a similar group share knowledge and experiences with each other. It involves autistic and neurodivergent people educating their peers, focusing on shared experiences, understanding, and mutual support. This approach is particularly valuable because it recognises that those with lived experience of neurodivergence are often best positioned to support and guide others facing similar challenges. Peer education empowers individuals by creating a sense of community, encouraging self-advocacy, and reducing isolation. It also challenges traditional top-down teaching models by placing neurodivergent voices at the centre. Peer education promotes autism acceptance through authentic, relatable exchanges, offering insight that clinical or outsider perspectives often miss.

Peer mentorship

Peer mentorship is a supportive relationship between neurodivergent individuals based on shared lived experiences. A mentor offers guidance, emotional support, and understanding to help their peer navigate challenges related to identity, social interactions, or daily life. Unlike traditional mentorship, this approach prioritises shared experience over hierarchical knowledge, creating a more empathetic and authentic connection.

For autistic people, such relationships offer an environment of mutual understanding, where the mentor and mentee connect on a level that promotes authentic self-acceptance and personal growth. Peer mentorship in neurodivergent communities is instrumental in helping individuals build confidence, reduce feelings of isolation, and develop coping strategies for navigating a neurotypical world. This model centres the value of community-driven support and the power of shared journeys in creating empowerment.

Periventricular nodular heterotopia

Periventricular nodular heterotopia (PVNH) happens when neurons fail to migrate properly during early brain development. Instead of reaching the brain's outer layer (the cortex), where complex thought, perception, and behaviour are processed, these neurons form nodules along the brain's ventricles – fluid-filled spaces that cushion and protect the brain.

This structural difference can cause epilepsy, cognitive variations, or sometimes no noticeable symptoms at all. PVNH often has a genetic basis, with variants in genes like FLNA playing a key role, especially in more severe cases. It is more commonly identified in cis females, who typically experience epilepsy as a primary symptom. In cis males, PVNH is often linked to more significant challenges, such as intellectual disabilities and congenital anomalies.

There is also a recognised connection between PVNH and conditions like Ehlers-Danlos syndrome, highlighting the overlap between neurological and physical health. Support for individuals with PVNH needs to be tailored and compassionate, recognising the varied ways it can present and impact daily life.

PVNH not only highlights the complexity of brain development but also challenges traditional notions of what is considered 'typical' versus 'atypical' neurology. These nodules highlight the substantial diversity in how brains are built and how they work. Instead of seeing PVNH purely as a medical condition, it can also be viewed as one of many ways that human brains adapt and function, even when development takes an unexpected route.

Person-first language ⚖️ 🚫

Person-first language refers to placing the person before the identity descriptor, such as saying 'people with autism.' This approach is controversial, as many autistic people prefer identity-first language, like 'autistic people,' which affirms neurodivergence as an inseparable and essential aspect of identity.

Person-first language can suggest that autism is undesirable, temporary, or something to overcome, which misrepresents its permanent and natural place in an individual's neurology. It also mirrors how negative states are often described, such as 'someone with cancer,' reinforcing the idea of autism as a condition to be 'carried' or 'cured.'

This perspective clashes with the neurodiversity paradigm, which views autism as a valid, lifelong variation in human experience. Identity-first language is widely seen as more empowering and aligned with the realities of autistic lives.

Personal Independence Payment (PIP) ⚖️ 🔵

Personal Independence Payment (PIP) is a UK government benefit aimed at helping disabled people, including autistic individuals, manage the additional costs of daily living and mobility challenges. Eligibility depends on how a disability affects 'daily functioning,' not on income, savings, or specific diagnoses. PIP has two components: 'daily living' and 'mobility,' each awarded at a standard or enhanced rate based on assessed support needs.

The PIP application process is often deeply stressful for autistic people. The paperwork demands extensive detail about daily struggles, which can feel overwhelming. Assessments frequently reduce lived experiences to checkboxes, forcing applicants to justify their need for support. This approach can feel dehumanising and invalidating, especially when assessors lack understanding of autism.

The process tends to focus on visible physical limitations while overlooking less obvious but equally significant challenges, such as communication, sensory processing, and executive functioning difficulties. Assessors also sometimes rely on brief observations during a single interview, failing to account for fluctuating needs where some days require far more support than others. These shortcomings can result in inaccurate assessments and unfair outcomes for autistic applicants.

Pervasive developmental disorder-not otherwise specified

Pervasive developmental disorder-not otherwise specified (PDD-NOS) was a diagnostic label used to describe individuals who exhibited autistic traits but did not meet the full criteria for other specific diagnoses. This term was part of the older diagnostic framework before being removed with the release of the DSM-5 in 2013, where it was absorbed into the broader category of Autism. PDD-NOS was often considered a 'catch-all' diagnosis, leading to confusion due to its vague definition. Its removal from diagnostic standards is significant as it aligns with the neurodiversity paradigm, which reframes autism as part of natural human variation rather than a collection of fragmented categories.

Phantom sensations

Phantom sensations refer to physical feelings or sensory experiences without an immediate external cause. An autistic person might feel a phantom touch, warmth, or tingling on their skin, reflecting unique sensory processing. These sensations arise from the brain's interpretation of sensory signals, illustrating the connection between interoception (the internal sense of one's body) and sensory processing differences.

While often linked to external physical stimuli, phantom sensations can also result from non-typical neurological wiring, where the brain amplifies or misinterprets sensory signals. They differ from mirror-touch synesthesia, where observing someone else being touched triggers a mirrored tactile response. In contrast, phantom sensations usually occur independently of visual cues and stem from the brain's internal sensory processing.

Phelan-McDermid syndrome

Phelan-McDermid syndrome (PMS) is a rare genetic condition linked to a deletion or mutation of the SHANK3 gene on chromosome 22. This gene is essential for neurological development and synaptic function. Individuals with PMS often experience developmental delays, speech difficulties, and motor skill challenges. Other common traits include low muscle tone (hypotonia), large hands, and distinctive facial features, though these vary. Seizures, sleep disturbances, and gastrointestinal issues may also occur.

A genetic test is the only definitive way to diagnose PMS. Its impact differs widely between individuals, emphasising the need for personalised support. Rather than focusing on 'normalisation,' care should prioritise enhancing quality of life and respecting each person's unique neurological identity.

Phonological process problems

Phonological process problems refer to difficulties that individuals have learning to speak specifically with regard to understanding the patterns of sound production and/or rules in speech. These issues occur when certain sounds or sound sequences are altered in ways that make speech less intelligible. In neurodivergent populations, phonological difficulties can emerge as part of the broader landscape of language differences, requiring an approach that is both accepting of neurodivergent communication styles and supportive of alternative methods of speech development. For example, autistic people may have unique ways of processing and producing speech sounds due to underlying neurological differences. Support may involve speech therapy that is neurodivergent-affirming and avoids pushing towards neurotypical norms.

Pica

Pica is the consumption of non-food items such as dirt, chalk, or paper. This behaviour is commonly linked to nutritional deficiencies, stress, or developmental differences. The most common types of pica include geophagia (eating clay and sand) and pagophagia (eating ice), the latter of which has been strongly linked to low iron levels. Approximately 12% of children have engaged in pica behaviour at some point in their lives, with pica prevalence peaking at 36 months and then decreasing with age. However, pica can be prevalent among autistic individuals due to sensory needs or as a response to anxiety. It is vital to understand that this behaviour as reflecting an unmet need and, as such, requires understanding and appropriate support. Effective management involves assessing environmental, sensory, and nutritional factors, identifying triggers, and offering safe alternatives. Collaboration with dietitians or occupational therapists can help create supportive strategies.

Polytropism

Polytropism refers to a cognitive style often linked with neurotypical individuals, characterised by the ability to shift focus across multiple tasks and engage with a wide range of activities simultaneously. This contrasts with monotropism, commonly associated with autistic individuals, where deep, singular focus on a specific interest is preferred. While polytropism supports broader, generalised attention, monotropism enables intense focus and detailed knowledge in one area. These patterns are not exclusive to neurotypical or neurodivergent people, as individuals may exhibit either style depending on context. The value in recognising polytropism lies in understanding that diverse neurological styles – whether monotropic or polytropic – each offer unique strengths.

Post-traumatic stress disorder

Post-traumatic stress disorder (PTSD) is a significant mental health issue that arises following exposure to traumatic events. For autistic people, PTSD can be more prevalent due to heightened experiences of sensory trauma and social rejection. Shutdowns, where stress energy is stored in the body, are a common trauma response in autistic individuals, reflecting the profound impact of unprocessed trauma. This trauma often manifests as severe anxiety, sleep disturbances, and persistent emotional distress. However, PTSD in autistic individuals can also manifest in subtle and less obvious ways, making it challenging to diagnose and address. One such manifestation is the 'fawn response,' which is a form of appeasement where an individual tries to pacify interpersonal threats by mimicking a safe state. This can be mistaken for genuine calmness, making it difficult even for professionals to recognise. Symptoms like emotional dysregulation, negative self-perception, and dissociation are also common yet often overlooked.

The lack of understanding and support for trauma in autistic people can exacerbate these conditions, leading to long-term psychological harm. Service providers working with autistic people who have PTSD must implement trauma-informed support systems that acknowledge and support their unique lived experiences.

IN MY OWN WORDS: JOAN LAPLANA

At the start of the COVID pandemic, I left my desk job as a senior staff nurse and was redeployed to work in the COVID intensive care unit (ICU) at my hospital.

Emotionally, I was hit very hard. Every day I went on a rollercoaster from joy to grief in a matter of seconds, experiencing anxiety, fear, insecurity, guilt, anger, and loneliness along the way. The work was often bleak, and I needed to constantly be on alert. I couldn't lower my guard for a moment because a single mistake could cause an unnecessary death.

Every time I opened the doors of the ICU, I knew I was risking my own life as well. There is a huge psychological pressure when you confront your own mortality, a constant voice whispering that you could be next.

We wore Personal Protective Equipment (PPE) constantly. All I could see were the eyes of my colleagues, and the connection and camaraderie we once relied on felt lost. It was stiflingly hot and sweaty throughout the 12-hour shifts, and I couldn't lift my visor to dry my face or take a sip of water. Breaks were carefully planned to eat, drink, and remove and replace PPE to use the bathroom.

Psychologically, I was not prepared to cope with the sheer volume of deaths and the intense pain we experienced daily. I often second-guessed the decisions I made during my shifts. Sometimes I was so anxious that I would call the unit afterwards to check on a patient, needing to know how they were doing.

I felt overwhelmed by the torrent of emotions. My only way to cope was to shut down my feelings entirely and block out the outside world.

But soon the cracks began to show. Broken nights piled up, and little by little, fatigue took over my body. Mood swings became more frequent, and one day, I had a panic attack at work. By the end of the second COVID wave, I was diagnosed with PTSD.

Looking back, I believe being autistic had a profound influence on how I experienced and managed – or failed to manage – my PTSD. Growing up, I mastered the art of masking, pretending everything was fine and bottling up my emotions to comply with society's expectations. This ingrained habit of hiding my true self made it harder for those around me to notice when I was struggling. I kept pretending everything was okay until I reached a breaking point. My inability to seek help or express my emotions contributed enormously to my mental health crisis.

However, receiving a PTSD diagnosis marked the beginning of a journey of self-discovery and acceptance. It taught me to recognise the toll masking had taken on my mental health and helped me realise the importance of being honest about how I feel. For the first time, I allowed myself to let go of the mask and express my emotions without the fear of being judged or singled out.

While my journey through PTSD has been painful, it has also been transformative. It has given me a deeper understanding of myself and the tools to face the future with greater authenticity and resilience.

Power of attorney

A power of attorney (POA) is a legal mechanism through which an individual (referred to as the 'donor') grants another person (the 'attorney') the authority to make decisions on their behalf. This arrangement is typically utilised when the donor cannot make decisions independently due to health issues, absence, or other reasons. POAs can cover financial matters, health, and care-related decisions, with powers defined by the specific terms of the agreement. The attorney is legally required to act in the donor's best interests, and their authority can be broad or limited.

POA frameworks vary globally. In the UK, key types include ordinary power of attorney, lasting power of attorney (LPA), and enduring power of attorney (EPA), each serving distinct purposes. Australia's system differs by state, with general POAs for financial matters and enduring POAs (EPOA) continuing after loss of capacity. India typically uses general and special POAs, mainly for financial and property affairs, with healthcare POAs being rare. In the US, POA laws vary by state, and similar diversity exists in other countries, reflecting local legal requirements and priorities.

Prader-Willi syndrome

Prader-Willi syndrome (PWS) is a rare genetic difference resulting from abnormalities in chromosome 15, affecting approximately 1 in 10,000 to 30,000 individuals worldwide. PWS is primarily characterised by issues with metabolism and appetite regulation, with individuals often experience a chronic feeling of hunger, leading to challenges around food intake and weight management.

PWS also involves cognitive, physical, and behavioural differences, including developmental delays, learning difficulties, and reduced muscle tone. These differences can shape an individual's interaction with their environment and community. People with PWS also often have a diminished sensitivity to pain, which can mask the severity of injuries, fractures, or infections. When alexithymia is also present, the difficulty in identifying or expressing physical discomfort may further complicate pain management.

Precrastination

Precrastination refers to the urge to complete tasks well ahead of deadlines, often to reduce cognitive load and alleviate anxiety about unfinished responsibilities. In ADHD individuals, it can stem from challenges with time perception, impulse control, and a fear of forgetting tasks. For autistic people, it may reflect a preference for structure and predictability, driven by a desire to minimise the uncertainty of incomplete tasks.

Although precrastination might seem productive, it often arises from underlying anxiety rather than genuine efficiency. This coping mechanism can sometimes lead to rushed work or increased stress. Further research is needed to better understand its effects on well-being and cognitive health.

Prejudice

Prejudice involves forming judgements about someone or something based on preconceived ideas, often without personal experience or factual evidence. It is rooted in stereotypes and can target ethnicity, gender, disability, or neurological identities such as autism. For example, it may arise when people assume that neurotypical ways of thinking and behaving are superior, which can lead to the marginalisation of neurodivergent individuals. This has been demonstrated many times in previous research where workforce professionals have been found to exhibit significant implicit bias against autistic individuals.

Prejudice is also driven by irrational fears. For example, one prevalent fear is that neurodivergent people might be 'faking' their diagnoses to gain special treatment, such as extra accommodations at school or work. This belief, referred to as the 'fear of the disability con,' contributes to widespread stigma despite research showing that such fakery is extremely rare.

Premenstrual dysphoric disorder

Premenstrual dysphoric disorder (PMDD) refers to a severe form of premenstrual syndrome (PMS) that includes intense emotional and physical symptoms. It is not simply 'bad PMS' but a serious condition that can deeply affect daily life, particularly during the luteal phase of the menstrual cycle. Symptoms include extreme mood swings, irritability, anxiety, depression, and physical discomfort like bloating or breast tenderness. While hormonally driven, PMDD's psychological impacts are significant and often misdiagnosed as other mental health conditions. Within neurodivergent communities, understanding PMDD is especially important due to overlaps with sensory sensitivities and emotional regulation difficulties. Autistic individuals, for instance, may already experience heightened emotional intensity or difficulty communicating distress, and the cyclical nature of PMDD can intensify these patterns, potentially leading to misinterpretation by healthcare providers.

Presuming competence ⚖️

Presuming competence refers to the fundamental belief that all individuals, including autistic people, possess potential and ability, even when they may not be able to communicate in typical ways or meet neurotypical expectations. This approach rejects the assumption of incapacity often placed on neurodivergent individuals due to their differences in communication, learning, or behaviour. Presuming competence is crucial because many autistic people, especially those with high support needs or who are non- or minimally speaking, are at risk of being underestimated especially by professionals and educationalists. This mindset shifts away from focusing on limitations and allows for richer, more empowering interactions, advocating for dignity, respect, and equal access to opportunities.

Procrastination 💬

Procrastination is the act of delaying tasks despite knowing there may be negative consequences. It is often misinterpreted as laziness or poor discipline. For ADHD individuals, it commonly stems from executive functioning challenges, such as difficulties with task initiation, working memory, and prioritisation. Autistic people may procrastinate when sensory overwhelm occurs or when specific conditions needed for task engagement are unmet.

A neurodivergent-affirming perspective reframes procrastination as a response to external and internal barriers rather than a personal flaw. Environmental mismatches, lack of structure, or anxiety-inducing situations frequently contribute to this behaviour. Procrastination often signals a misalignment between task demands and an individual's cognitive patterns. Addressing it effectively requires tailored support, reduced stigma, and an understanding of diverse working styles.

Professional stigma 🌿 🚫

This type of stigma refers to negative attitudes and assumptions held by professionals, often within health and social care and education, about neurodivergent individuals, including autistic people. Such stigma is often rooted in outdated understanding and knowledge, influenced by the medical models that pathologise autism and disability. As a result, professionals may unintentionally perpetuate ableist attitudes. This kind of stigma can manifest during the any element of interaction, from assessment through to the delivery of support. Overcoming professional stigma requires a shift towards the neurodiversity paradigm, where autism is seen as a valid identity, and professionals work in partnership with autistic people to meet their needs in a respectful, supportive manner. Working within a workplace culture that promotes, validates, and leverages neurodivergent identities among professional staff is also vital.

Profound and multiple learning disability

Profound and multiple learning disability (PMLD) refers to individuals who face both significant cognitive and physical disabilities. It reflects the intersection of profound learning challenges with complex physical and sensory needs, affecting communication, mobility, and self-care. Communication passports are a valuable tool for supporting people with PMLD. These documents record personalised communication styles, helping carers and professionals understand and respond to non-verbal cues such as gestures or body language.

People with PMLD often need highly specialised and consistent support to engage with their surroundings and participate in daily activities. Effective and compassionate care shifts the focus from limitations to recognising and nurturing each person's unique ways of learning and interacting. This approach ensures that people with PMLD have the fullest opportunity to thrive and express their individuality.

Proprioception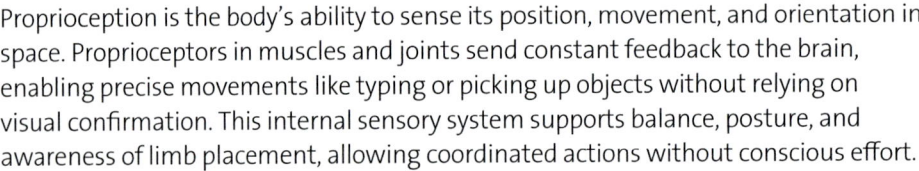

Proprioception is the body's ability to sense its position, movement, and orientation in space. Proprioceptors in muscles and joints send constant feedback to the brain, enabling precise movements like typing or picking up objects without relying on visual confirmation. This internal sensory system supports balance, posture, and awareness of limb placement, allowing coordinated actions without conscious effort.

For autistic people, proprioception often functions differently, potentially leading to sensory challenges. Some may experience heightened or reduced proprioceptive sensitivity, which can affect motor coordination or the ability to gauge the amount of force necessary to perform tasks. For example, people with proprioception issues may lean on objects to gain additional tactile input, compensating for the lack of internal sensory feedback and helping them feel more secure and grounded. These differences can also result in clumsy movements or difficulties with activities such as writing or balancing.

Prosody

Prosody is about the patterns of speech, such as how our voice rises and falls, how fast or slow we talk, and how we stress certain words. It helps convey emotion and meaning beyond just the words themselves. For example, if someone says, 'I'm fine,' with a flat tone, it might sound like they are upset, even though the words suggest they are okay. This is prosody at work.

Autistic people may use or interpret prosody differently, affecting how they are perceived in social interactions. These differences are not a lack of communication ability but a variation in expression and experience. An autistic person might speak in a monotone or with intonation patterns less common among neurotypical speakers, leading to misunderstandings about their emotional state. They may also struggle to convey sarcasm or subtle meanings through prosody, which can result in social or professional misinterpretations. In neurodivergent-affirming spaces, these differences are recognised and accepted.

Prosopagnosia

Commonly referred to as 'face blindness,' prosopagnosia is a neurological phenomenon that affects a person's ability to recognise faces. This can impact day-to-day social interactions, as those with prosopagnosia may struggle to identify familiar people, even close friends and family members, based solely on their facial features. Instead, individuals with prosopagnosia might rely on alternative cues such as voice, clothing, or specific habits to recognise others.

Prosopagnosia exists on a spectrum, ranging from mild difficulty to a complete inability to recognise faces. It can cause feelings of shame or embarrassment, reducing confidence and motivation in social or professional settings. Anxiety, sensory overload, or mental fatigue can worsen the difficulty, especially in overstimulating environments or during periods of low energy.

Both neurodivergent and neurotypical people can experience prosopagnosia, but it appears more frequently in autistic individuals due to differences in visual processing, social perception, and a higher likelihood of anxiety or non-accommodating environments.

Pseudobulbar affect

Pseudobulbar affect (PBA) is a neurological phenomenon characterised by sudden, uncontrollable episodes of laughing or crying, which may not correspond to an individual's actual emotions. It frequently occurs in people with neurological conditions or injuries that impact how the brain regulates emotion, such as multiple sclerosis, Parkinson's, or traumatic brain injury. PBA's emotional outbursts can lead to embarrassment, social isolation, and misinterpretation by others. Increasing awareness and understanding is key to reducing stigma and ensuring those affected receive appropriate empathy and support.

Pseudothymia

Pseudothymia describes a form of profound openness and honest engagement in social communication, particularly evident among autistic individuals. This concept goes beyond the typical notion of gullibility, capturing a unique and deeply sincere way of interacting with others that often lacks filters for deceit, hidden agendas, or social manipulation. Pseudothymia highlights a willingness to take others at face value, often leading to more authentic interactions but also potential vulnerability in social contexts shaped by dishonesty or subtext. The phenomenon reflects a dedication to truth and genuine connection yet can be challenging when navigating a world that rewards subtlety, deception, or hidden motives.

Psychological well-being

Psychological well-being is the state in which an individual feels balanced, content, and mentally resilient. For autistic and other neurodivergent people, psychological well-being often hinges on feeling accepted in settings that understand and respect their neurological differences. Well-being in this context is not about 'fitting in' with neurotypical norms but about thriving in an inclusive environment that respects diverse ways of thinking and communicating, allowing the individual to be their authentic self without needing to mask.

When autistic individuals embrace their identity and feel connected to a supportive community, they experience improved quality of life, reduced feelings of loneliness, and greater mental resilience.

As such, well-being does not simply mean the absence of anxiety or depression but the active presence of an environment and relationships that affirm one's neurodivergent identity and enable safe and meaningful connectedness with their communities.

Psychosis

Psychosis describes a state of disconnection from reality, often involving experiences such as hearing, seeing, or sensing things that others do not (commonly called hallucinations), or holding strong beliefs that may seem unusual or illogical to others (sometimes called delusions). These experiences are often accompanied by intense emotions and a profound shift in how a person understands or relates to the world around them.

Importantly, what is termed *psychosis* may be experienced and understood in a range of cultural and personal ways. The World Health Organisation and United Nations have both advocated for a shift away from narrow biomedical models — which frame psychosis purely as an illness of the brain — and towards trauma-informed, rights-based, and socially-contextual approaches to mental distress. These models prioritise compassion, autonomy, and an understanding of mental health that takes social, economic, cultural, and historical context into account.

Stigma surrounding psychosis continues to be a serious issue. It frequently leads individuals and families to hide their experiences, which delays access to meaningful support. Contrary to common and harmful stereotypes, people experiencing psychosis are far more likely to harm themselves than others. The idea that they are dangerous is not only false — it increases their vulnerability by fuelling discrimination, coercion, and exclusion.

Psychosis is not a condition in itself but a description of certain experiences that can arise in various contexts — including trauma, stress, extreme sleep deprivation, grief, and a range of health and life events. It can affect both neurotypical and neurodivergent people.

Neurodivergent people — including autistic individuals — may be more vulnerable to mental distress such as psychosis, not because of their neurology, but because of factors like systemic oppression, sensory trauma, social exclusion, or unmet communication and support needs. This highlights the urgent need to build communities and systems that offer compassionate, non-judgemental, and human rights–driven support — not just for individuals, but for families and society at large.

Public stigma 🌿 🚫

Public stigma refers to the negative stereotypes, discrimination, and misconceptions imposed by society and the general public on individuals or groups. Public stigma creates and reinforces inaccurate and harmful ideas that autistic and neurodivergent people are deficient, disordered, need 'treatment,' and of less inherent value for society than neurotypical people. This stigma is perpetuated by social, cultural, and medical institutions that fail to understand or accept neurodivergence.

The impact of public stigma is profound, leading to marginalisation, ostracism, exclusion, misunderstanding, internalised ableism, and the denial of appropriate support or respect for neurodivergent individuals. Addressing public stigma is challenging but possible. It involves a long-term process of shifting societal and cultural attitudes to focus on acceptance, promoting positive representations, and educating people about the value and legitimacy of neurodivergent identities. However, even with education, biases towards autistic people can persist at an unconscious level. This is because while training and education can improve conscious understanding and social interactions with autistic people, deep-seated stereotypes often persist unconsciously. Addressing this requires ongoing, active engagement beyond basic training. Integrating autistic voices into education and workplace cultures, challenging media stereotypes, and enabling continuous exposure to diverse autistic experiences are also critical strategies for long-term change.

Pupil referral units

Pupil referral units (PRUs) in in the UK provide alternative schooling for young people unable to attend mainstream schools. Despite their intended supportive role, concerns persist about their effectiveness and inclusivity, particularly for neurodivergent students, including autistic individuals. Autistic students are over-represented in PRUs, often placed there due to behaviours linked to unmet sensory or communication needs rather than intentional disruption.

Exclusion rates have risen in recent years, increasing demand on PRUs, creating long waitlists, and straining financial resources. Critics argue that these units operate within a system that frames behavioural divergence as problems to be 'fixed' rather than differences to be understood. Supporting neurodivergent students effectively requires rethinking the frameworks governing PRUs, focusing on meeting diverse neurological needs instead of enforcing behavioural conformity.

R

Reasonable adjustments ⚖️ 🛡️

Changes in environments, processes, or expectations to ensure fair access and participation for neurodivergent people can be considered 'reasonable adjustments.' This is crucial as societal structures are almost always designed by neurotypicals for neurotypicals, and as such, society can 'disable' neurodivergent people. Therefore, adjustments should remove or, at the very least, minimise these barriers, promoting fairer inclusion.

For example, an autistic employee might benefit from flexible working hours to manage sensory sensitivities or additional time to process tasks. Organisations implementing appropriate adjustments for neurodivergent employees often see significant productivity gains.

The Reasonable Adjustments Passport is an innovative tool that documents agreed-upon adjustments, ensuring consistent support even when roles or managers change. This concept aligns with the social model of disability, which emphasises that the environment must adapt rather than expecting the neurodivergent individual to conform.

Regressive autism 💬 🚫

The term 'regressive autism' is often used to describe a phenomenon where an autistic child, previously appearing to develop social or communication abilities in a manner comparable to neurotypical children, undergoes a noticeable change involving the loss or reduction of these skills, typically between the ages of 1 and 3 years. However, the term itself is deeply negative and stigmatising. Autism is a neurological identity, not a condition that can 'regress' or deteriorate; framing it as such perpetuates a pathologising narrative rooted in the medical model of disability. The term implies a negative transformation or decline, when, in fact, these changes are not a decline per se but rather an adaptive neurological shift or as a response to sensory, environmental, or developmental differences.

DOI: 10.4324/9781003477297-15

Rejection sensitivity dysphoria 💬 🌿

Rejection sensitivity dysphoria (RSD) involves heightened emotional responses to real or perceived rejection, often stemming from past trauma associated with rejection. Individuals with RSD may experience overwhelming feelings of anxiety, sadness, or anger when they believe they have been rejected, criticised, or have failed in some way, even when the rejection may seem minor or unintentional to others.

This sensitivity can manifest physically, with some describing rejection as a visceral sensation, like being punched in the stomach. Neutral social cues, such as a friend's lack of laughter at a joke, might also be misinterpreted as rejection.

To avoid this emotional pain, individuals with RSD may adopt people-pleasing behaviours, striving to meet others' expectations at the cost of their own well-being. Over time, this pattern can lead to burnout, isolation, and strained relationships, as perceived slights may trigger withdrawal or heightened emotional responses.

IN MY OWN WORDS: IQRA BABAR

In my case, RSD is one of the most prominent ADHD traits that I have and continue to experience. For me, RSD feels like one of two things. It will feel like a sudden crash wave of emotions flooding over me, which I have little control or grip over. Other times, it feels like a bottle slowly filling itself up with doubt, concerns, and small inconveniences that accumulate until the bottle is tipping over, on the verge of explosion. It is full of small changes in micro-expressions, or very minor inconveniences that convince me that the other person loathes my existence and wishes they never had anything to do with me.

The worst part is that no matter how often I experience it, I still plead guilty to falling for these feelings. Paintings my brain paints of false external perceptions of myself are, in my eyes, easy to believe. This is likely due to the immense bullying I experienced during my time in school, and the aftermath is still felt today, which is perhaps expressed and felt through my sensitivity towards the idea of being rejected by others. My RSD is intense. The feelings never feel 'less than' whenever I experience it. The feeling of (potentially) being rejected, especially by those you love, admire, or appreciate is a suffocating one that clogs up your ability to reason. I guess you could say that RSD is an incredibly emotional experience with the unpredictability of where a trigger of fear perception may appear and how the RSD might present itself.

> The intensity of my RSD most likely stems from the bullying I endured from peers growing up, especially in high school. It has also had a detrimental effect on how intensely I overthink social situations, to the point where I will go into meltdown, unable to process the 'what-ifs' of situations I do not have clarity on. The constant bombardment of rejection and 'fake friendships' from others has morphed me into someone deathly afraid of it and anxious of not being good enough for that person for them to reject me and perceive me negatively. I had gone through a plethora of episodes growing up where I had to endure fake friendships or people manipulating me easily due to me being over-trusting of people too quickly, which is something I still struggle with today. The anxiety surrounding a person's intentions is something I find difficult to process and understand today but am working towards making it easier for myself so that I am less hard on myself.
>
> I still struggle as an adult in regulating myself to manage my RSD as it's such an intense, isolating experience. But I think that's normal, and it's okay to not necessarily know all the answers regarding how to manage it or understand it fully. It's taken me this long to understand the hows and whys of my RSD, and even then, sometimes I slip up in understanding it, because the experience can, at times, happen so fast, or something that feels so rapid out of nowhere, but in actuality, it's an accumulation of so many stimuli.

Repetitive behaviours

Repetitive behaviours are often misunderstood. Far from being negative or problematic, these actions are usually essential self-regulation tools that help autistic people manage and interpret an overwhelming world. They can include physical movements like hand-flapping or rocking as well as verbal repetitions of phrases.

Despite their importance, these behaviours are frequently mislabelled as symptoms of a 'deficit' or 'disorder.' Harmful therapies, such as applied behaviour analysis (ABA) or positive behaviour support (PBS), often attempt to suppress or eliminate them, reflecting the flawed belief that autism is something to be 'corrected.'

The term itself is also problematic, as 'repetitive' carries negative societal connotations. A more respectful term would be 'stimming behaviours' or 'self-regulatory behaviours,' which better reflect the purpose they serve for autistic people.

Resilience

Resilience is the psychological capacity to cope with and recover from difficulties and challenging circumstances.

The development of resilience involves not only relying on one's internal resources but also involves seeking support from the community, friends, and family. Helping other people can also boost one's own resilience, as can practicing mindfulness, such as deep breathing and meditation, which promote calmness and reduce stress. However, resilience and developing a 'thick skin' are often temporary solutions. Real change requires a societal shift towards inclusivity and non-ableist structures. In such a world, autistic individuals would not need to rely on resilience just to exist; they could thrive without constantly depleting their energy ('losing spoons') to manage unsupported environments.

Championing resilience should not overshadow the importance of acknowledging and addressing times of vulnerability. Not everyone will feel resilient all the time, and that is okay. Societal expectations to constantly exhibit resilience can be harmful, leading individuals to mask their true feelings to avoid the stigma of not being resilient and reduce the likelihood of accessing the support they need. Therefore, encouraging open expression of emotions without fear of judgement is key.

IN MY OWN WORDS: KOSJENKA PETEK

"Resilience is not a DIY effort" read an article title I came across. The article delved deeply into the critical role of external support systems. Shouldn't that be common knowledge by now, in the 21st century? Isn't it something parents and teachers should instil early on – that we need external support systems, nurturing environments, and just the right amount of frustration to help us thrive and build resilience? Surely, we all know this by now?

We have the research. We have the understanding. And yet, we still expect independence, a growth mindset, resilience, and personal strengths to magically manifest in a crying baby, a child, or a young adult. You can sense my frustration, can't you?

In Croatian society, we glorify perseverance and teach ourselves to forgive our mistakes through fire and hell, believing it will lead to resilience. It's practically a badge of honour. Or, depending on how much therapy you've had, transgenerational trauma.

But without providing the environment, the infrastructure, and the support that traumatised, stigmatised, and marginalised minorities need, asking for resilience is like trying to fix an aortic tear with a band-aid.

As an autistic woman, a teacher, and a mother, I want us to talk about true resilience – not the kind that rewards the trauma and stress of masking or forces us to endure discomfort without meaningful support.

What does it mean to be truly resilient? How much healthy frustration does it take? Who gets to decide? What's at stake?

For me, it's always come down to the people in my life who saw me for who I was, who stretched out a hand, and who gently guided me. I call it stretching my comfort zone. When I'm in safe, trusting hands, I find I can go beyond my wildest dreams. Once I experience that sweet spot of growth a few times, I feel ready to face the world – to walk into a tough situation, attend a doctor's appointment, make a phone call, or even drive a car on my own.

For my autistic child, it took a village: my girlfriends, other neurodivergent women, autism professional allies, and compassionate, humane teachers. Together, they helped him move past his traumatic experiences and start building resilience – at the age of 15. It's nothing short of a miracle that we managed it in only a decade.

What makes a difference, alongside timely and high-quality support, is psychoeducation. Most of us are cognitively able to receive adapted psychoeducation – learning about our disabilities, our strengths, our areas for growth, and how to navigate relationships and the wider world. This includes setting boundaries and respecting others'.

When I think about resilience, I'm struck by how interconnected and challenging it is for us. For someone who grows up without resilience, helping them develop it later is a long and often lifelong process. Sometimes I doubt whether a person who missed out on timely support can ever lead the same trusting and fulfilled life as someone who had a steady hand to guide them.

As a society, we still haven't created the necessary support systems or systemic environments to foster resilience for all. And that leaves me wondering: how many more people could lead happier, more fulfilled lives if we made this one of our priorities?

Resource-based schools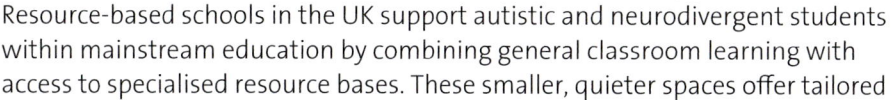

Resource-based schools in the UK support autistic and neurodivergent students within mainstream education by combining general classroom learning with access to specialised resource bases. These smaller, quieter spaces offer tailored academic, sensory, and therapeutic support without fully separating students from their peers.

Students move flexibly between mainstream classes and the resource base according to their needs, with some requiring occasional support and others more regular access. Highly trained staff, including SENCOs and therapists, collaborate to address individual strengths and challenges, while sensory-friendly spaces help reduce sensory overwhelm.

Although well-established in the UK, this structured and standardised model remains relatively uncommon internationally.

Rett syndrome

Rett syndrome is a complex neurodevelopmental phenomenon, predominantly impacting girls, with an estimated prevalence of 1 in 10,000 female births globally. It emerges in presentation after an early period of seemingly typical growth, usually between 6 and 18 months of age, as children begin to lose the ability to speak, walk, and control hand movements. These shifts include gestures like hand-wringing as well as challenges with muscle coordination. Despite its connection to a genetic mutation on the MECP2 gene, Rett syndrome is rarely passed down through families, with most cases resulting from new genetic mutations. It has also been historically been misclassified as an autism-related diagnosis even though it is a separate phenomenon.

Rhizomatic communities

Rhizomatic communities refer to groups that form and develop in a non-hierarchical and decentralised manner, much like the underground root system of a rhizome, where connections can be made in numerous directions without a single central point of control. In fields like medicine, this approach is evident in the free open access medical (FOAM) education community, where professionals share resources like blogs, podcasts, and infographics, emphasising collective knowledge over individual authorship. This model empowers participants to continuously refine and adapt the information based on real-time feedback, creating a constantly evolving knowledge base that is particularly valuable in fast-paced, information-rich environments.

For neurodivergent people, rhizomatic communities are particularly valuable as they enable diverse voices, perspectives, and lived experiences to coexist, intersect, and inform one another without the imposition of a rigid structure. This model of community reflects the neurodiversity paradigm itself, which values a plurality of ways of thinking and being. These communities are fluid, adaptable, and resistant to exclusionary practices, allowing individuals to create meaningful, organic connections based on shared experiences of difference and mutual support.

S

Safe spaces 🛡

Safe spaces are environments designed to protect neurodivergent individuals, including autistic people, from discrimination, judgement, and harm. These spaces prioritise acceptance, respect communication differences, and accommodate sensory and social preferences, offering a refuge from neurotypical societal expectations. Safe spaces also support individuals to replenish their energy or 'spoons' after sensory, social, or demand overload.

Safe spaces are also key elements of a neurodivergent-affirming, inclusive workplace. By carefully managing factors like acoustics, lighting, and colour schemes, workplaces can significantly enhance employee productivity and well-being. For instance, using low-stimulant colours and avoiding patterns helps create a calming environment, while acoustic dampening materials reduce disruptive noise, which can be a key distraction for autistic people. The inclusion of sensory-friendly zones – such as quiet areas or flexible spaces for activities like stretching – can provide essential breaks from overstimulation, boosting focus and reducing stress. Lighting design also plays a critical role, with the use of high-quality LEDs to avoid flicker and glare.

The home should also serve as a vital safe space for neurodivergent individuals. By adapting elements such as lighting, sound, and physical layout, homes can be personalised to meet sensory needs. Simple changes like reducing clutter, using soft lighting, or creating quiet corners can provide much-needed comfort and security, ensuring that the home remains a sanctuary from external pressures.

Saviour syndrome 🚫

Saviour syndrome refers to a problematic mindset where non-autistic individuals position themselves as 'rescuers' of autistic people, often assuming they know what is best for them. It is rooted in the belief that autistic people need saving, promoting a narrative that devalues their autonomy and lived experience. Savior syndrome often manifests through well-meaning actions that ignore the actual desires, needs, and voices of autistic individuals. Such behaviour can lead to paternalism and perpetuate harmful stereotypes, reinforcing the idea that autistic

DOI: 10.4324/9781003477297-16

people are inherently 'broken' or in need of external intervention to lead meaningful lives. Instead, autistic people need others to respect their autonomy and support to enable their self-determined goals without imposing external ideals or assumptions of what their life should be. As such, true support lies in acceptance and respect, not in being a 'saviour.'

Schizophrenia and schizoaffective disorder

Schizophrenia and schizoaffective disorder have traditionally been understood as psychiatric or mental health conditions, often characterised by experiences such as hallucinations, delusions, and altered perceptions of reality. Schizoaffective disorder combines these features with significant mood disruptions, including depression or mania. Both phenomena typically emerge later in life, usually in adolescence or early adulthood.

However, some advocates and researchers are pushing to expand the neurodiversity framework to include schizophrenia. This broader view acknowledges that schizophrenia involves differences in how individuals process information, interact socially, and perceive the world – elements often associated with neurodivergence. This evolving perspective challenges the medicalised framing and helps to reduce the stigma by instead focusing on creating more compassionate and inclusive environments than solely focusing on direct treatment.

Scripting

Scripting is when autistic individuals rehearse or repeat dialogue from movies, books, or conversations, often to prepare for social interactions. It serves as a valuable tool for navigating complex or unpredictable situations. By relying on familiar, pre-learned scripts, they can feel more secure in unpredictable environments.

Scripting is not limited to spoken words; it can also include mimicking tones, phrases, or body language. Scripting can provide comfort, aid self-regulation, support emotional processing, and serve as a form of self-expression.

It also plays a key role in gestalt language acquisition, where individuals learn larger chunks of language – such as phrases – rather than single words. Over time, these chunks are broken down and personalised, contributing to more flexible speech patterns.

Selective mutism

Selective mutism refers to the experience of individuals, often children but also adults, who are able to speak in some settings but find themselves unable to do so in others, particularly in situations where speaking is expected. It affects about 1 in 140 children under the age of eight years and is frequently misunderstood as stubbornness or refusal. In reality, it stems from intense anxiety, often social or sensory, which makes speech feel impossible in specific environments.

This difficulty is not a choice but a response to overwhelming stress. It can significantly impact education, friendships, work, mental health, and overall life opportunities.

Selective mutism may be more common among multilingual children. This is because the stress of navigating different languages, especially in unfamiliar environments, can further increase anxiety around communication.

The term 'situational mutism' is sometimes used to describe similar experiences. However, it is generally considered synonymous with selective mutism. Both terms refer to the same underlying phenomenon, though 'selective mutism' is the widely recognised and diagnostically accepted term.

Reducing anxiety through safe, accepting spaces allows individuals to express themselves more freely without fear or pressure. Selective mutism should not be stigmatised or viewed as a flaw. Instead, it deserves understanding, respect, and supportive approaches that honour the individual's experience.

Self-acceptance

Self-acceptance is a crucial concept for neurodivergent individuals, involving a profound and ongoing journey of understanding and embracing one's authentic self. It often reduces the need to mask, improves mental health, and strengthens belonging – especially when supported by neuro-affirming communities. Aligning with one's neurological identity, rather than striving to meet neurotypical standards, brings peace and empowerment.

The process often entails reflecting deeply on personal experiences, distancing from societal pressures, and re-evaluating past events. It involves practising self-compassion, setting boundaries, and celebrating one's unique strengths and challenges. This journey can be significantly supported by neuro-affirming support from others, especially within autistic and neurodivergent-led spaces and communities. Unconditional encouragement from family and friends further reinforces progress. Therapy with autistic mental health professionals or experts in autistic identity can also be highly effective.

Challenges arise when self-identification or diagnosis happens later in life, or when internalised ableism, stigma, and poor mental health are present. Societal stigma, lack of resources, and limited access to autistic-led, neuro-affirming therapies can further hinder self-acceptance.

Voices of Neurodiversity

IN MY OWN WORDS: JOAN LAPLANA

If you asked me 10 years ago if I was autistic, I would have laughed in your face. It was my ex-wife was the first person who told me that I might be autistic when I was on my late 30s. I completely dismissed the idea.

Because of my unconscious bias, I thought when people talked about autistic people were referring to people like Raymond Babbit from the famous film *Rain Man*. I thought that autistic people did not talk or interact with anyone. I thought that autistic people lacked empathy, had limited social skills, and were emotionally cold, and unimaginative. That was not my case. I had a job and a family; I was part of society.

How wrong I was. I always felt different. I am very creative. I always have many creative ideas, most of them admittedly useless, but I was stuck in a traditional and task-orientated workplace where I felt I couldn't be myself or express any of my ideas. On a few occasions that I tried it but that did not end well and often managers isolated me and invited me to find another job. Because of that, I felt emotionally drained. I could also say that my own self-care was compromised.

In 2018, I was diagnosed with depression. Looking back, I think I was misdiagnosed. I am convinced I had an autistic burnout. It was also then when I had decided to explore the possibility of me being autistic. The journey has not been easy. Initially I felt very vulnerable and fragile. It didn't help that some of my colleagues, despite my diagnosis, still did not believe me. If I had a penny for every person that told me that I must be wrong because I do not look autistic, I would probably be millionaire by now.

But it was not until after the COVID pandemic and I was diagnosed with PTSD that I finally began to fully embrace the reality that I was autistic. And it was thanks to the work with my therapist that I realised that I do not need fixing. Being autistic is part of who I am and there is nothing wrong with me. Since then, I have become an autistic public figure, and I have openly disclosed my diagnosis. But it has been a long journey of discovering and acceptance that I could not have done without the support of my therapist and other coaches.

Self-advocacy ⚖️ 🛡️

Self-advocacy refers to the process by which autistic people assert their own needs, preferences, and rights, often in settings where their voices have been historically marginalised. It is about having autonomy and taking control of one's life, making decisions regarding personal support, education, or health and care. Autistic self-advocates promote understanding of autism from an insider's perspective, countering harmful stereotypes and misconceptions, such as viewing autism through a deficit-based lens. As such, it is a powerful form of resistance against societal ableism, a way to reclaim autonomy and challenge exclusionary practices.

It goes beyond simply speaking up for one's own needs; it is about actively reshaping environments, policies, research studies, and cultural narratives to reflect the diverse ways in which autistic people experience the world. In practice, self-advocacy has led to profound shifts – whether by autistic individuals influencing public policy, reshaping education systems to accommodate diverse learners, or rejecting harmful therapies that enforce neurotypical standards. It transforms not only individual lives but also community-wide understandings of acceptance and belonging. The heart of self-advocacy is empowerment, as autistic people increasingly lead movements that dismantle systemic barriers and demand authentic representation and inclusion.

Self-harm

Self-harm involves intentionally causing physical injury to oneself, often as a way to manage overwhelming emotions, anxiety, or distress. For autistic and other neurodivergent individuals, it can stem from sensory or demand overload, internalised ableism, stigma, discrimination, loneliness, or external stressors – especially in persistently unaccommodating environments.

Rather than being a deliberate attempt to end one's life, self-harm often serves as an emotional and psychological survival strategy. Yet, tragically, suicidal ideation and suicide rates remain significantly higher within the autistic population compared to the general population.

Addressing self-harm in neurodivergent individuals requires moving beyond judgement to focus on understanding its roots. Creating accepting, sensory-friendly, and safe environments, alongside providing affirming and non-coercive emotional support, is essential in reducing reliance on self-harm as a coping mechanism.

Self-medication

Self-medication involves using substances – such as alcohol, prescription drugs, or illicit substances – to manage mental or physical health difficulties without professional guidance. While it may offer temporary relief, it often leads to addiction, worsened health issues, and increased dependency.

Autistic individuals are particularly vulnerable to self-medication, often due to limited access to appropriate, neurodivergent-affirming support. Many mainstream services lack autism understanding, resulting in long waits or ineffective care. Some research indicates higher rates of substance misuse among autistic people compared to non-autistic populations, highlighting the urgent need for timely, tailored mental health and substance use support.

Prevention remains more effective than treatment. Inclusive and equitable socio-cultural settings, particularly in education and employment, can significantly improve autistic mental health and well-being, reducing reliance on self-medication. Valuing and accepting autistic individuals, rather than subjecting them to exclusion or discrimination, is crucial in addressing the root causes behind these harmful coping strategies.

IN MY OWN WORDS: ANDREW KINGSLOW

Takes deep breath . . .

Where do I begin? So, we have to start with the autistic outsider syndrome. I never felt a part of a conversation, nor did I have a close group of friends. I was habitually bullied and spent a lot of my formative years trying to be what I thought people wanted me to be as opposed to developing my own sense of self.

Turns out, I learnt quite quickly that, for me, the effects of alcohol, for instance, immediately increased my confidence, my ability to make eye contact and engage, and gave me a sense of belonging within my peer groups. More than anything, alcohol blurred the edges of a life spent on the edge of sensory overload.

The problem with that is I've always been extreme in my endeavours, so it would be quite natural for me to take to drinking in an extreme way. I think it stems from my inability to identify my feelings particularly well.

I am quite heavily involved in the music industry, so it was only a matter of time before I found myself being offered more illicit contraband. The problem with this was that, whilst all of my colleagues bounced off the walls, I had my "Neo in the Matrix" moment – my thoughts became more linear, I was genuinely interested in what people had to say, and if anything, and possibly also quite dangerously, I felt less neurodivergent.

This is where self-medication enters the room.

Self-medication really became a code word for addiction for me. Like with any medicine, prolonged use requires higher doses, and the dependence eventually erodes freedom and confidence, replacing them with apathy and anxiety.

I read that autistic people are nine times more likely to become addicted to drugs. This really resonated with me and led me to seek help through therapy.

If I'm being honest, I do believe there are potentially positive effects that can be extracted from certain psychotropic drugs, as current research suggests. I truly hope future generations can benefit from such trials. The problem we face as the neurodivergent community is that there isn't a safe way to access these now, and we certainly aren't in a position to moderate and control the things that give us momentary relief from the stresses of life.

Self-regulation

Self-regulation empowers neurodivergent people, especially autistic individuals, to manage overwhelming sensory and emotional input. It is not about behavioural 'control' but rather about using adaptive strategies to restore neurological balance and maintain well-being. This deeply personal process honours an individual's natural sensory and emotional rhythms, promoting resilience and self-acceptance.

Autistic people self-regulate in many ways, such as through stimming – like hand-flapping – or by retreating to sensory-safe spaces. Deeply absorbing interests also provide stability, offering predictability and a calming focus. These strategies create a vital buffer against chaotic or intrusive environments, safeguarding autonomy, comfort, and emotional equilibrium.

The time required for self-regulation varies greatly, depending on the intensity of sensory overwhelm, energy reserves (or 'spoons'), and whether the environment feels safe and accepting. This process should never be rushed or interrupted.

Self-stigma

Self-stigma occurs when autistic individuals internalise society's negative perceptions and misconceptions about autism. This internalisation can lead to feelings of undeservingness, isolation, or shame about one's identity. For many, self-stigma develops after prolonged exposure to stereotypes and discrimination. Its effects are significant including the increased risk of mental health problems, masking, and reduced self-worth and self-efficacy. It can also result in self-exclusion, with individuals avoiding autistic communities due to difficulty accepting their diagnosis or fear of association with other autistic people. Safe, neurodivergent-affirming spaces that encourage authentic expression and self-acceptance can be powerful tools in addressing this.

While related, self-stigma and internalised ableism have distinct focuses. Internalised ableism reflects society's broader negative views of disability, often causing individuals to feel pressured to 'overcome' their needs, measure themselves against neurotypical standards, or hide their differences. Self-stigma, however, is more specific – it emerges when someone internalises shame or negativity about their neurodivergent identity, often triggered by direct discrimination or negative feedback. While internalised ableism reflects a broad acceptance of ableist standards, self-stigma represents a focused response to personal stigmatising experiences.

Stigma-protection and resistance interventions can help autistic and neurodivergent individuals reject self-stigma. However, the most effective – and most challenging – approach is addressing and eliminating social stigma at its root.

SEND Code of Practice ⚖️ 🏢

The SEND Code of Practice aims to secure tailored, holistic support for young people with special educational needs and disabilities (SEND), framing their educational rights in the UK. While its guidance mandates that local authorities and schools engage collaboratively with families, seeking to address each young person's unique educational, health, and social needs, in practice, the Code often falls short of these ideals. Families frequently navigate an uphill battle for the support promised by law, facing inconsistent implementation due to limited resources and staff shortages.

The Code is also criticised for its adherence to deficit-based views on SEND, where young people's needs are addressed primarily as barriers rather than as facets of diverse identities. As such, the SEND Code stands at a crossroads between well-meaning policy and the need for a more inclusive, genuinely collaborative practice.

Sensory assessments 🛡️

Sensory assessments help identify how an autistic person processes sensory input, which often differs significantly from typical experiences. These assessments, often conducted by occupational therapists and sensory specialists, not only identify sensory sensitivities such as hypersensitivity (over-responsiveness) or hyposensitivity (under-responsiveness) to stimuli like noise, light, touch, taste, or movement, but they also delve into how well a person integrates multisensory information, such as combining sight and sound.

These assessments can uncover subtle sensory processing differences that are not captured by traditional diagnostic tests, providing a deeper understanding of an individual's sensory experiences. They guide recommendations for adjustments at home, school, or work to align environments with sensory needs. Informal sensory assessments conducted by autistic individuals or their families can also help identify and address sensory challenges. Since sensory profiles can change, periodic reassessments ensure ongoing relevance and effectiveness.

There are also some emerging technologies that are revolutionising sensory assessments, offering real-time and more precise methods for understanding sensory processing differences. Tools such as wearable devices and virtual reality, for example, provide new ways to monitor physiological responses and simulate sensory environments, respectively. This integration of technology not only enriches the assessment process but also promotes a more personalised approach to sensory support, making it easier to adapt environments to the unique sensory needs of each individual.

Sensory avoidant

Being sensory avoidant refers to autistic and other neurodivergent people making a deliberate effort to reduce or avoid certain sensory experiences. This is often a response to experiencing heightened sensory sensitivity, which can encompass a wide range of sensory inputs such as sounds, lights, textures, or smells. For example, an individual might find the hum of fluorescent lights or the feel of certain fabrics overwhelming and may avoid environments where these are present. Being sensory avoidant is not inherently a problem or a 'disorder' but rather a natural response to an environment that is not supportive of their sensory needs. It is about managing sensory input in a way that ensures comfort and reduces anxiety.

Sensory crisis

A sensory crisis refers to a state of overwhelming sensory overload experienced by some autistic people when their environment becomes too intense or chaotic for their sensory processing systems. This could result from an excess of sensory input such as loud noises, bright lights, or strong smells. A sensory crisis can be acute, occurring suddenly in response to immediate sensory overload, or chronic, where an ongoing, persistently overwhelming environment leads to prolonged distress and sensory fatigue. During a sensory crisis, an autistic person might experience extreme distress, which could manifest as physical reactions like covering ears or eyes, repetitive movements, or withdrawing from the environment to seek calm. It is vital to understand that such reactions are not behavioural 'outbursts' but rather necessary coping mechanisms in response to a sensory environment that is unbearable for the individual.

Sensory gardens

Sensory gardens are purposefully designed spaces that engage the senses, offering a therapeutic and calming environment for autistic individuals and those with sensory sensitivities. These gardens feature elements like textured plants, aromatic flowers, and soothing water features, providing opportunities for sensory exploration that can be stimulating or calming, depending on individual preferences.

These gardens create inclusive environments where neurodivergent individuals can engage with nature at their own pace. By incorporating quiet zones, shaded areas, and thoughtful seating arrangements, sensory gardens help reduce sensory overload, support emotional regulation, and promote overall well-being.

Sensory integration

Sensory integration is the brain's process of organising and interpreting sensory input from both the environment and the body. This includes traditional senses (sight, hearing, taste, touch, smell) as well as the vestibular (balance) and proprioceptive (body position) senses. For autistic and other neurodivergent individuals, this process often involves navigating sensory hypersensitivity or hyposensitivity, which can make the world feel overwhelming or underwhelming.

Sensory experiences play a central role in daily life, influencing social interactions, emotional regulation, and comfort. Sensory rooms offer controlled environments designed to support sensory integration by providing stimuli tailored to an individual's sensory profile. These may include tools such as bubble tubes, fibre optic lights, or interactive projections. Other sensory tools like weighted blankets, tactile wall panels, noise-cancelling headphones, sensory putty, and fidget toys can help with self-regulation, reduce anxiety, and improve sensory processing. Personalisation is key to ensuring these supports effectively meet individual needs.

Sensory overload

Sensory overload occurs when the brain is overwhelmed by more sensory input than it can process. Autistic individuals often experience heightened sensitivity to stimuli like sounds, lights, textures, smells, visual activity, pain, or proprioceptive challenges. This can be intensely painful and exhausting, sometimes leading to meltdowns, shutdowns, self-medication, or even self-harm, particularly when mental health is strained or energy reserves are depleted.

Managing sensory overload involves understanding a person's sensory profile to tailor environments to their needs and build resilience in challenging situations. Strategies include creating sensory-friendly spaces or quiet rooms and planning to minimise exposure to overwhelming stimuli. Offering compassionate, non-judgemental support is essential in helping individuals cope with sensory overload.

IN MY OWN WORDS: ANDREW KINGSLOW

All my life, I have suffered from sensory overload, often without realising it. As a child, it was frequently mistaken for sulking or being antisocial. However, on reflection, I now recognise behaviours like hiding in a dark room during large family gatherings as clear signs of sensory overload. One particularly traumatic sound was that of a vacuum cleaner. The loud, droning noise would have me clutching my ears and hiding under the bed as a small child. Even now, I can often be seen with my fingers in my ears on the tube, as the sound of metal scraping against metal feels almost bone-breaking to me.

I've always been sensitive to loud sounds, and certain noises have a physical, almost tangible effect – I would even compare the sensation to pain. Just thinking about those situations can evoke a similar response as I write this.

My sensitivity isn't limited to auditory overload; it extends to textures as well. Materials like velvet, cotton wool, and similar fabrics send shivers through my body. To be honest, I can't even look at such materials without feeling uncomfortable.

As an adult, social situations like public and networking events are particularly challenging. The ambient noise, the sea of faces, and the overwhelming energy drain my masking abilities and, consequently, my energy reserves. I often retreat to a corner or feel the need to leave entirely. Since I no longer drink, these situations feel even more difficult; alcohol once provided an analgesic effect that made them more bearable.

In the workplace, I've discovered a new form of sensory overload. When colleagues deliver information too quickly or in a way I don't fully understand, I struggle. I also find it difficult to interpret tones of voice, which causes me to a) become anxious, b) shut down, or c) become defensive or combative. In these moments, I can literally feel my blood starting to boil as confusion takes over.

To manage sensory overload, I've learned to limit the time I spend in crowded, noisy environments. My noise-cancelling earphones are my saviour, helping me block out overwhelming sounds and providing a much-needed sense of calm. They are an essential part of my daily life and allow me to function in situations that would otherwise be unbearable.

Have I experienced meltdowns due to sensory overload? Definitely. However, I've learned to recognize the signs and do my best to avoid situations that could trigger them. With tools like my noise-cancelling earphones and better awareness of my limits, I've found ways to make life more manageable.

Sensory processing differences vs sensory processing disorder

The term 'sensory processing disorder' is not recognised within the neurodiversity paradigm as it does not align to view that sensory differences are a natural variation in the human experience and integral aspects of an individual's identity. Rather, the concept arises from the medical model, categorising sensory sensitivities as deficits that need 'treatment.' However, sensory processing differences are not disorders to be fixed but are valid variations that should be supported, understood and respected. This is why those aligned to neurodiversity and the social model of disability adopt the term 'sensory processing differences' rather than 'sensory processing disorder.' By using 'differences,' the emphasis shifts towards acceptance and the need for supportive environments that respect these variations. This approach encourages a supportive framework that values individual sensory profiles and promotes the inclusion of all sensory experiences as valid and significant aspects of human diversity.

Sensory rooms

Sensory rooms are carefully designed spaces offering sensory inputs such as lights, sounds, textures, and smells to support individuals, including autistic people, who benefit from sensory regulation. These spaces aim to help users calm or stimulate their senses in alignment with their unique sensory profiles.

For sensory rooms to be effective, they should be co-designed with input from those with lived experience of sensory processing differences. This ensures the spaces meet individual needs and avoid the pitfalls of a generic, one-size-fits-all approach. Adaptability is key to addressing the highly individualised nature of sensory needs.

Ideally, sensory rooms would be standard in schools, workplaces, and high-stress environments like airports and sports stadiums. However, their availability remains limited. Quick, easy access is essential to prevent sensory crises from escalating into meltdowns or shutdowns. While safety measures are necessary, reducing bureaucratic barriers is critical to ensuring timely access.

Sensory seeking

This term refers to behaviours exhibited by some neurodivergent people who actively seek out sensory experiences to fulfil their unique sensory needs. This might include enjoying strong tastes, engaging with bright lights, or seeking deep pressure sensations. Such behaviours are not signs of dysfunction but of a different sensory processing system that the environment may not be fully aligned with.

For example, individuals with interoception differences, who may struggle to recognise or regulate internal bodily states like hunger, thirst, or fatigue, often compensate by seeking external sensory input. Engaging with spinning objects, bright lights, or loud sounds can provide consistent and predictable feedback, helping them manage internal states and achieve a sense of calm or balance. These external sensory experiences serve as grounding tools, enhancing bodily awareness and self-regulation.

Sensory-specific satiety

This refers to the natural decrease in appetite or satisfaction for a specific food as it is consumed, which plays a critical role in dietary variety and regulation of overall food intake. This effect is usually more pronounced for the food being eaten than for other available foods, which explains why someone might feel full from a meal but still desire dessert or differently flavoured foods.

For autistic individuals, this phenomenon can present in unique ways due to sensory sensitivities. Imagine an autistic child who adores the texture and taste of smooth mashed potatoes but finds the sharpness of a tomato sauce overwhelming. They may eat large amounts of the mashed potatoes without feeling the usual decline in appetite because their sensory system finds it comforting and predictable. However, the introduction of even a small dollop of tomato sauce could abruptly shift their sensory experience from pleasant to unbearable, making it impossible to continue eating.

Conversely, some autistic people may grow tired of even their favourite food halfway through a meal, as their sensory system quickly becomes overstimulated by the repetition of taste or texture. These differences illustrate how sensory-specific satiety, far from being a simple appetite mechanism, can deeply interact with the sensory world of an autistic individual, shaping their eating habits in unexpected ways.

Sensory synergia

Sensory synergia refers to the experience where an individual's sensory environment perfectly aligns with their unique sensory processing preferences, leading to enhanced cognitive performance and overall well-being. This state highlights how sensory inputs can significantly influence mental clarity, creativity, and problem-solving. Unlike sensory overload, which can cause distress, sensory synergia epitomises the optimal alignment of external stimuli with one's sensory needs, producing an empowering and invigorating experience. This harmonious state can vary in duration, from brief moments to several hours. However, sustaining sensory synergia can be challenging, as it often requires adjustments to one's sensory environment.

IN MY OWN WORDS: AGUSTINA CARDOSO

For me, sensory synergia is like unlocking a hidden level of consciousness, a secret room within my mind where everything is heightened yet harmonised. It's a state of relaxed alertness, like finally finding a calming and cosy place in the middle of a city.

Normally, my mind is a whirlwind of thoughts, sensations, and perceptions. There's always something to process, analyse, and react to, colours and sounds constantly shifting and vying for attention. But in these moments of sensory synergia, that internal noise fades away and it's replaced by a sense of clarity and serenity.

It's not just an external experience, though. I don't just look more comfortable and at ease. Internally, my thoughts have slowed down; worries and anxieties are replaced by a sense of peace and well-being.

This state of sensory harmony isn't something I can always achieve on demand. It often arises spontaneously, triggered by specific combinations of sensory input. For instance, after a long day at university, overwhelmed by sensory overload, I've developed a routine that often brings about this sense of synergia.

I come home and immediately change into comfortable clothes and set up warm lighting to counteract the hours of blue light I've been exposed to. Then, I put on my noise-cancelling headphones and lose myself in my favourite video game on my Nintendo Switch. From an outsider's perspective, it might seem like I'm isolating myself from the world. And in a way, I am, but I see it less as isolation and more as me creating my own little world within the walls of these sensory regulating activities.

This self-created world allows me to not only rest and recharge, but to truly come back to myself. This deliberate crafting of my sensory environment allows me to filter out the noise and find that inner peace, that sense of synergia where my mind and body feel truly in tune.

Sensory synergia is a reminder that our senses are not just passive receptors of information but active participants in shaping our thoughts, emotions, and experiences,` and what we do to regulate them can play a significant key role in our well-being.

Sensory trauma 💬 🚫

Sensory trauma refers to the distress and psychological impact that can result from intense or overwhelming sensory experiences. It emphasises how sensory environments can profoundly impact mental and emotional well-being, especially when those experiences are intense, prolonged, or unavoidable.

For autistic individuals, who process sensory input differently, understanding sensory trauma is essential. Many have heightened sensitivity to stimuli like sounds, lights, or textures. Environments that clash with their sensory needs can trigger immediate crises, such as meltdowns – outward expressions of intense distress – or shutdowns, where they withdraw entirely to cope. Repeated exposure to such environments can lead to sensory trauma, resulting in chronic anxiety, discomfort, and even physical pain. This enduring impact underscores the necessity of creating sensory-friendly spaces to support the well-being of neurodivergent individuals.

Shutdown

Unlike a 'meltdown,' which is more outwardly expressive, a shutdown is characterised by withdrawal and reduced responsiveness. This is because a shutdown involves the person being temporarily unable to engage with their environment due to overwhelming sensory, emotional, or cognitive demands. It is, therefore, a protective psychological mechanism because the withdrawal allows the individual to mitigate any further overload by retreating and disconnecting from external stimuli.

Shutdowns may manifest as silence, immobility, or minimal interaction and can last from minutes to hours or even days. They are not signs of unwillingness or negativity but are essential coping strategies. They are more likely in environments that lack neuro-affirmative support, where masking, suppressing one's true self, or a lack of understanding adds strain. Shutdowns also become more likely when mental energy or resilience (often referred to as 'spoons') is depleted.

The onset of a shutdown can be gradual or sudden and might go unnoticed, even by the person experiencing it, particularly if they struggle with interoception. This lack of awareness can increase anxiety and impact psychological well-being.

Six-second rule

The six-second rule is a strategy that can be used during communication with neurodivergent people and can be particularly valuable for autistic individuals. This practice revolves around consistently allowing at least six seconds – and often more – for someone to process and respond during interactions. The approach counters the dominant pace of neurotypical conversations which often favour rapid responses. By intentionally pausing, the rule allows for varying processing speeds and encourages authentic exchanges without pressure. The concept helps to challenge the incorrect assumption that immediate responses equate to attentiveness or capability.

Social anxiety 🌿 👥

Social anxiety is a complex and multifaceted experience, often characterised by an intense fear or discomfort in social situations. Among autistic individuals, social anxiety is particularly common, with some studies indicating a lifetime prevalence of up to 80%. It can manifest as heightened sensitivity to social scrutiny, a pervasive worry about being judged, or an overwhelming fear of negative evaluation. It is distinct from general shyness and can deeply affect relationships, education, and employment. Neurodivergent individuals, particularly those with challenges in social communication or sensory processing, face unique difficulties. For example, an autistic person might find eye contact overwhelming or experience heightened anxiety in noisy environments due to sensory sensitivities. These experiences increase fears of being judged or misunderstood because neurotypical expectations often fail to account for such realities. This creates a vicious cycle, where anxiety about being perceived as 'different' or 'awkward' worsens the condition and makes social situations even harder to navigate.

Social capital 👥 💧

Social capital refers to the networks of trusted relationships and connections that individuals can safely rely on for emotional and psychological well-being. For neurodivergent people, particularly autistics, it is crucial in addressing social isolation and preventing both emotional and social loneliness. Social capital can save lives by reducing the risk of suicide, as supportive networks act as a buffer during mental health crises.

Neurodivergent-led spaces and communities are vital in creating this kind of support. These environments provide a sanctuary where individuals experience a genuine sense of belonging – a 'tribe' where they can be their authentic selves without pressure to mask or conform. Within these spaces, people share experiences and challenges, learn from one another, and feel valued.

Building social capital not only strengthens these connections but also helps reduce internalised ableism and stigma. However, barriers such as stigma and lack of accessible spaces often prevent individuals from forming the connections they need. This highlights the importance of creating inclusive and supportive communities that ensure everyone has the opportunity to build meaningful social capital.

Social communication 👥

Social communication refers to the nuanced ways individuals exchange information and interact in social settings. It includes spoken and non-speaking methods such as facial expressions, body language, eye contact, tone of voice, and implied meaning. Studies indicate that over 90% of social communication occurs without speech.

For autistic individuals, social communication often differs from neurotypical patterns. These differences are not deficits but reflect the diversity of human communication. Autistic people may require more time to process conversations or rely on less conventional methods, such as body language or augmentative and alternative communication (AAC).

Cultural norms further shape communication styles, expectations, and pressures. Rules about who speaks first, the importance of eye contact, or emphasis on certain topics can pose additional challenges, particularly for demand-sensitive individuals, adding complexity to social interactions.

Social exclusion 🚫

Social exclusion is a profound challenge, particularly for autistic individuals, who often encounter significant barriers in forming and maintaining friendships and relationships. This exclusion frequently occurs in spaces dominated by neurotypical norms, where differences in communication and social interaction are misunderstood, undervalued, and unsupported. Non-affirming environments may unfairly label autistic people as aloof, disinterested, or unintelligent, leading to isolation and marginalisation.

The effects of social exclusion on mental health and well-being are profound. A lack of safe social spaces and inclusive relationships increases the risk of anxiety, depression, and loneliness. By contrast, neurodivergent-affirming environments that offer genuine inclusion create belonging, acceptance, and emotional security.

Social fatigue 👥 🌿

Social fatigue refers to the exhaustion autistic and other neurodivergent people may experience from navigating social situations, which often require sustained mental effort and adaptation. This fatigue arises because of the considerable mental processing needed to decode social cues, manage sensory inputs, and respond in ways expected by non-autistic peers. Unlike general tiredness, social fatigue is uniquely tied to the sustained effort of social engagement, particularly in environments that lack understanding or support for neurodivergent needs.

For example, an autistic teenager might experience social fatigue after a day at school, where they must constantly adjust their behaviour to meet neurotypical expectations. The toll of interpreting peers' shifting tones, suppressing natural stimming behaviours to avoid judgement, and enduring the sensory overload of bustling hallways and fluorescent lights can be immense. By the time they reach home, they may feel drained – not just physically tired but emotionally and mentally spent. Even a simple question, such as asking about their day, might feel overwhelming. Recovery from this level of exhaustion could require hours or even days of solitude, underscoring the profound impact of navigating environments that do not allow them to fully be themselves.

Social hangover

Social hangover describes the lingering exhaustion and emotional depletion that can occur after social fatigue. Unlike the typical sense of tiredness that might follow social activities, a social hangover is more profound, involving both physical fatigue and cognitive strain. This phenomenon highlights the significant effort required for autistics and other neurodivergent people to navigate social norms, process sensory input, and engage in communication, which may not come naturally to them.

Social hangovers underscore the need for recovery time after social engagements, including solitude and downtime, reflecting the intensive mental and emotional resources expended. It also reinforces the importance of creating supportive environments that minimise sensory and social overload.

Social model of disability

The social model of disability contrasts sharply with the medical model of disability. The medical model views disability as an individual problem, focusing on impairments or diagnoses. It implies that disabled individuals are 'broken' and need to be 'fixed,' 'treated,' or 'cured' through medical interventions. For example, the medical model would say an autistic person struggles in a shopping supermarket due to their autistic neurology.

Alternatively, the social model argues that disability arises from societal barriers. It locates 'disability' externally, in systemic barriers, derogatory attitudes, and social exclusion. For instance, an autistic person might find shopping at supermarkets difficult not because they are autistic, per se, but because these environments are not designed to support their sensory needs. Thus, society actively 'dis-ables' individuals by not catering to their diverse characteristics.

Developed by UK disability rights activists in the 1970s and 1980s, the model has laid the groundwork for significant legislative changes in disability globally mandating reasonable adjustments to remove barriers and promote equality, such as the Disability Discrimination Act of 1995 and the Equality Act of 2010 in the UK. The model aligns well with the neurodiversity paradigm, which recognises all forms of neurological development as equally valid and valuable. It emphasises the importance of acceptance and inclusion rather than trying to change or 'normalise' neurodivergent people.

IN MY OWN WORDS: ADITI GANGRADE

When my partner and I first began to suspect that we might be neurodivergent, like many others, we instinctively turned to the internet for answers. We hoped to find guidance or clarity about autism and ADHD, but what we encountered in India was disheartening and, quite frankly, disturbing.

Instead of supportive resources or understanding, the search results were filled with medical professionals touting so-called 'cures.' Even more alarming were the suggestions on how to 'detect' autism in the womb to prevent giving birth to an autistic child. It was shocking to see the extent of misinformation and the number of dangerous, unverified treatments preying on parents' fears. These so-called 'therapies' not only exploited vulnerable families but also caused real harm to neurodivergent children.

In India, religious leaders – 'babas' – play a huge role in misleading families. They offer false promises of 'removing' autism from children, while some doctors promote harmful treatments like stem cell therapy despite it being banned by the National Medical Commission of India.

I actually directed a film to raise awareness about the dangers of stem cell therapy for autism and developmental and intellectual disabilities. It's horrifying how common these stories are – parents receive their child's diagnosis as if it's the end of the world. They're told that their 'normal' life is over, and that autism is a problem that will ruin everything.

In some families, especially joint ones, the mother often bears the brunt of this news. She's blamed and harassed by her in-laws for giving birth to a 'defective' child. Neurodivergence, and the struggles that come with it, are dismissed as excuses. Families face societal judgement, unsolicited advice, and even ostracization. So, when a medical professional offers a 'cure' or a quick fix through corporal punishment or unverified therapies, many families jump at the chance, desperate for any solution.

While the disability rights movement in India has gained momentum in the last decade, it has rarely focused on developmental and intellectual disabilities. This leaves a gap in awareness and acceptance of neurodivergence.

And I've seen doctors promoting their centers with videos claiming miraculous improvements – autistic kids making eye contact or ADHD kids forced to sit still through any means necessary.

In India, two kinds of people tend to hold the most trust: babas and doctors.

The reason the social model of disability hasn't taken root here is because of our collectivist culture. Herd mentality prevails. People don't want to understand why you're different – they just want you to conform.

Here, systems come first, and people are expected to fit into them rather than the other way around.

Explaining the social model of disability to people has been an uphill battle. I've had people say things like, "But you don't even look autistic," or "Would you say that about cancer? Should we 'affirm' cancer too?"

That's one of the reasons we started using our platform to educate and entertain people about social issues. Growing up, I was often made to feel like my neurodivergent traits were character flaws. I was told things like, "If you don't make eye contact, people will think you lack confidence." That phrase alone haunted my childhood and teenage years. And don't even get me started on, "If they can do it, why can't you?"

I blamed myself for everything. I even reached a point where I felt so worthless that I became suicidal.

I took classes to improve my communication, self-esteem, and impulsive behaviors, trying to 'fix' myself. Then, I met my partner – someone who was like me and accepted me as I was. He admired me and my work, and that acceptance was the turning point. I started believing in myself again.

Together, we've since educated medical professionals, corporate leaders, media professionals, and parents on the social model of disability. We do it through workshops, films, and content. Our platform, Much Much Spectrum, has made the social model a norm for many around the world.

The social model of disability is rooted in human rights – it recognizes that disabled children and adults aren't the ones who need 'fixing.' Instead, it's society that needs to evolve to be more inclusive.

And here's where the magic happens: when the social model meets science, real progress becomes possible.

The social model means understanding that when an autistic child has a meltdown, they aren't throwing a tantrum – they're communicating. It's about validating their experience rather than trying to punish or correct it.

At the same time, science helps deepen our understanding of child development, brain function, and growth. When these two approaches intersect, we get a powerful combination that transforms how we support neurodivergent individuals.

As I've continued on this journey of self-discovery, I've sought out a community in India. Amid all the misinformation, I've also encountered wonderful, affirming doctors – those who embrace the social model of disability. These professionals aren't pushing cures. They understand that the real work lies in creating environments that are accessible, supportive, and respectful of neurodivergence.

Social Services and Well-Being (Wales) Act 2014

The Social Services and Well-Being (Wales) Act 2014 establishes a framework for social care delivery in Wales that centres on well-being, individual rights, and personal outcomes. It aims to promote independence and ensure care is tailored to each person's needs and circumstances. The Act requires local authorities to assess the needs of both adults and carers, enabling a more holistic support system. Collaboration among service providers and preventative measures to reduce future dependency on care services are central to its approach.

However, criticisms have arisen around its implementation, particularly regarding resource allocation and variable consistency across regions. Budget constraints and challenges in ensuring equitable care have undermined its effectiveness. Efforts to improve integrated care pathways and make services truly person-centred continue, but coordination remains a significant challenge.

Social stories

Social stories are visual tools that help autistic individuals navigate social situations by providing clear and structured information. They are typically presented as illustrated narratives that outline events or activities in sequence, offering step-by-step guidance. For example, a story about going to the airport might include images of the car ride, the airport, security checks, and boarding the plane. Social stories have expanded over time to cover diverse scenarios and formats, including videos, comic strips, and virtual reality.

These tools reduce anxiety by making situations more predictable and manageable. They are especially useful for autistic individuals who may feel heightened stress in unfamiliar environments. Social stories are also valuable for people with speech and language difficulties or visual learners. By offering information in an accessible format, they enhance understanding and comfort.

IN MY OWN WORDS: ADITI GANGRADE

Stories have the incredible power to change people.

My grandma would read me a bedtime story every night, and most of them had a moral. That was my first experience with social stories. She told me tales where girls broke stereotypes, where the protagonists made choices that went against what society expected of them.

Those stories shaped me more than I realized at the time.

My next encounter with social stories was during a roadshow, which is where I met my partner. We bonded over our shared love for listening and storytelling. Together, we traveled to 17 cities across India, documenting the lives and experiences of young people. We chronicled stories of mental health, exam pressure, gender identity, climate change, queerness – stories that reflected the real struggles of India's youth.

It was through this journey that my partner and I grew even closer.

Since then, we've created many films that tell stories like these. But I've realized that, in today's world, people are drowning in information. There are countless platforms, creators, and media companies. Information is accessible at all times, and we can connect with anyone from anywhere. Yet, despite all this access, Gen Z still grapples with loneliness, mental health struggles, and the feeling of not being understood.

In this age of content overload, what stands out is meaningful content that makes important issues engaging and relatable. This is something many young people are actively seeking.

But what do social stories mean for autistic people?

As an autistic person, I crave predictability. Unpredictable situations can feel overwhelming and confusing. For instance, when I meet new people, I like to know who I'm going to meet, what their name is, what they look like, and what we'll be talking about. Having that information helps me feel at ease, and thankfully, my team understands and accommodates these needs.

Every time we have a meeting with someone new, my team shares their social media profiles with me in advance so I can familiarize myself with them. We also go into every meeting with a clear agenda. It's an ideal way for me to work because it not only reduces anxiety but also helps me conserve energy for the things that truly matter.

I remember a time when my extended family had planned a picnic, and one of my younger cousins was refusing to go. His parents, and pretty much the entire family, forced him to join, and he was in a bad mood the whole way. To help calm him, I started explaining what we'd be doing at the picnic, which games we'd play, and even showed him pictures of the park. Gradually, I could see him relax.

This is what people often miss: every behavior has a reason. Yet, words like 'spoiled,' 'misbehaved,' or 'lazy' get thrown around so carelessly, especially by adults trying to label children or young people.

When I was a kid, comics and picture books were my escape when I was feeling low. They gave me a sense of comfort, and honestly, I think I've learned more about life and people from comics than I have from real-world interactions. When my mom was expecting my younger brother, I remember reading comics about what happens in a hospital and what it's like when a new baby joins the family.

Of course, reality turned out to be a bit different, but those books helped prepare me. I recall reading a story about a child who was bitten by an insect, so I knew right away that it was my job to protect my baby brother from bugs!

In the same way, the absence of good role models was something I felt deeply as a child. I've always learned better by watching someone do something, so I often think that if I had more positive role models growing up, I might have found my purpose – and myself – much earlier in life.

Societal stigma

Societal stigma refers to the widespread societal attitudes and beliefs that negatively stereotype and discriminate against autistic people. This stigma can lead to social isolation, invalidation, and fear of judgement. Many autistic individuals internalise these negative perceptions, resulting in shame, guilt, and self-blame. Stigma amplifies the challenges they face, often discouraging them from seeking support or sharing their experiences, which profoundly impacts mental health and well-being. It manifests as 'felt stigma,' where stigma is perceived and internalised, and 'enacted stigma,' where discriminatory actions are directly experienced. Both are deeply harmful. Stigma is also culturally specific, varying across communities and cultures.

While autistic and other neurodivergent people may have various support needs – such as speech and language support, sensory support, support with structured and predictable environments, and help in creating routines – the most crucial support need is always acceptance by families, communities, and society. Acceptance enables the fulfilment of other support needs and lays the foundation for autistic people to lead happy, healthy, and fulfilling lives. Reducing and eliminating societal stigma is therefore essential to achieving this.

IN MY OWN WORDS: IQRA BABAR

The perception of others about you is something easily feared amongst all neurodivergent folk, particularly those who possess an intersectional identity. The idea that others perceive you and that you have little control over their perception of you is scary enough. Having to live or work amongst it is a different story, and it is something I have experienced a lot growing up and even into adulthood.

Growing up, I was always perceived as the 'weird' kid. Looking back on it now as an adult, the auDHD traits are clear to me in my behaviour with others and habits I used to have. I would be called weird for being hyperactive or stimming externally with movement or vocally. It was isolating to be labelled 'weird' or 'strange,' or simply looked at differently to others. I hated being looked at 'differently' or to be considered 'different' in any capacity, as the connotation was usually negative, and in my case, it almost always was. Asking for help was something I struggled to do as I was anxious about being gaslit by peers, which did happen on a few occasions, both in primary and high school, so I learnt to keep to myself, enclosed in a shell of myself, which made high school a very isolating experience.

An incident which I will very briefly explain but will always vividly remember is being hated by a girl so much to the point where I was targeted by 50 peers in the year group, including her, to apologize to her for, in my eyes, attempting to stand up for myself, which it was. In the girl's eyes, however, it was unacceptable and I owed her an apology because I was always in the wrong and never her. This form of gaslighting stayed with me up till year 13 and made social interactions difficult. To this day, I struggle to not be hard on myself for my struggles as an auDHDer. It is a massive unlearning process that will take its time due to being engraved in the thought that everything somehow must be my fault. High school was extremely unkind.

The negative perceptions of me during high school escalated rapidly in the first year and resulted in me high-masking for the next 5 years up until 6th form, where my mask would slowly unravel due to the pressures of my Year 12 and Year 13 BTEC courses. When I got my autism and ADHD diagnosis at 17 years old, one of the biggest challenges I endured was the aftermath of confiding in my friends and how they perceived me. The best friends who I still have today wholeheartedly accepted me for me, regardless of my struggles and traits that differed me from the neuro-normative person. Others, on the other hand, started to perceive me differently, with negative connotations.

My ex-best friend, who behaved quite neutral when I had first confided in her, started to treat me more stand-offishly soon after, to the point where, when I was having a mentally bad day once, I was told to "stop blaming everything on my autism." This immediately told me that there was no level of understanding or empathy coming from her to me when it came to things that I struggled with or were out of my control. I felt negatively perceived and stigmatised as a 'liar.' She, along with a few others, at some point would ask me several times if I "really was autistic," and I can only assume it is because I am a Muslim, Pakistani woman and not a White male caricature.

Societal stigma and media representation are intersectional issues that go hand in hand more often than not. Back then, the quality of neurodivergent media representation was quite scarce, especially for anybody who looked like me. Because of this and the inadequate knowledge we are taught in schools, people will naturally form a 'stereotypical' perception of certain groups. This happened in my case, and it was difficult to deal with, mostly because I didn't know how to. I was confused about whether I should believe their perception of me, despite it making me feel isolated and singled out, but bullying does that to you. It's almost as if you gaslight yourself into thinking the other person is right about you more than you are about yourself. Such is the impact of stigma and negative perceptions of neurodivergent folk. It is already difficult to navigate in a capitalist-drenched society that was not built for us in any capacity, to manage how others perceive you to avoid being singled out due to behaviours out of your control makes it 100x harder.

Somatic alexithymia 💬

Somatic alexithymia refers to difficulties in recognising and describing physical sensations, particularly those related to illness or discomfort. It relates to the broader concept of alexithymia, which involves challenges in identifying and expressing emotions, but focuses specifically on physical rather than emotional experiences.

For autistic people, who often process sensory input differently, somatic alexithymia can complicate understanding and managing physical health. Struggles to identify sensations like pain or fatigue may lead to delayed healthcare or difficulty communicating needs.

Support strategies include using wearable devices like smartwatches or health monitors to track metrics such as heart rate, activity, and sleep. Sensory-mapping tools, such as apps for logging sensory and physical responses, can help identify patterns and detect signs of illness or pain early. Regular check-ins with trusted friends, family members, or competent healthcare professionals can also help.

Special Educational Needs and Disabilities 🏢

In the UK, Special Educational Needs and Disabilities (SEND) is the standard term used in education and public services to describe learning needs and disabilities requiring tailored support. SEND replaced the older term SEN (Special Educational Needs), which focused on learning difficulties without explicitly addressing disabilities. The change reflects a more inclusive approach. For autistic children, SEND highlights the need for accommodations like sensory, social, or communication support, without framing these needs as deficits or disorders.

Critics argue that SEND is rooted in a medical model of disability, focusing on individual challenges rather than environmental barriers. Instead, SEND frameworks should prioritise flexible, adaptive educational environments that support all learners, shifting from rigid developmental standards to an emphasis on acceptance and practical support.

Internationally, similar terms vary by country. The United States uses 'Special Education' and IEPs (individualised education programs) under the Individuals with Disabilities Education Act (IDEA). Canada refers to 'Special Education' or 'Exceptional Learners,' while Australia and many EU nations follow their own inclusive education guidelines.

Special Educational Needs and Disability Act 2001 ⚖️

The Special Educational Needs and Disability Act 2001 (SENDA) was a landmark UK law that strengthened the rights of students with special educational needs and disabilities (SEND). By amending the Education Act 1996, SENDA prohibited discrimination in schools and higher education and required institutions to make reasonable adjustments to support disabled students. These adjustments included tailored support services and modifications to improve accessibility. However, there was criticism that SENDA did not go far enough in mandating proactive inclusion, leaving gaps in support and accountability that later acts have sought to address.

SENDA's impact extended well beyond its time, reshaping educational practices and laying the groundwork for laws like the Equality Act 2010 and the Children and Families Act 2014. These acts built on SENDA's principles, further embedding disabled individuals' rights into the legal framework.

Its legacy remains significant, influencing how institutions strive for inclusive education and ensuring the needs of all learners are recognised and supported.

Special Educational Needs Coordinator

In UK schools, the Special Educational Needs Coordinator (SENCO) ensures students with special educational needs and disabilities receive effective, inclusive support. Their role focuses on managing resources and policies rather than providing direct assistance. SENCOs oversee Education, Health, and Care Plans (EHCPs), a legal framework outlining the support required for students needing alternative provisions. Despite this, EHCPs are often inconsistently implemented, leaving families to seek additional support or pursue legal action to secure their rights.

Approaches to supporting these students differ internationally. In the United States, Individualised Education Programs (IEPs) define tailored goals and supports, implemented by special education teachers and service providers rather than a single coordinator like the SENCO. Finland integrates SEND support directly into mainstream classrooms, with special education teachers collaborating closely with students and class teachers. Australia combines individual learning plans with input from both Learning Support Coordinators and classroom educators, reflecting a more collaborative, distributed model of support.

Special interests

The term 'special interests,' often replaced with 'dedicated interests,' describes the intense and passionate engagement that autistic and other neurodivergent individuals have with specific subjects or activities. This deep focus is not a trait to be 'managed' but rather a vital aspect of one's identity. Recognising the cognitive, emotional, and social advantages of these interests is essential, as they provide comfort, structure, and a rich avenue for learning and developing expertise. By valuing and supporting these pursuits, society can benefit from the unique insights and skills neurodivergent individuals bring, which, when nurtured and respected, can grow communities and the wider society.

Historically, 'special interests' have been framed within clinical discourse, often casting them as atypical or symptomatic behaviours. This is why the term 'dedicated interests' is preferred within the neurodiversity framework as it removes this pathologising undertone and, instead, emphasises the natural diversity in how people experience and express enthusiasm.

IN MY OWN WORDS: IQRA BABAR

It can be a pretty vulnerable action for me to open up to somebody about my interests, as the fear of rejection, being ignored, or somebody simply not caring is something that often looms over me. To unmask in front of anybody is a vulnerable action, and when I do, it is an incredible representation of trust from me to the other person. As a teacher with many interests in history, it feels rewarding to be able to share clusters of knowledge with others, even if they do not necessarily know how to respond but wholeheartedly take the time to listen to me. It makes me feel important, valued, and loved. Many of my friends will constantly reassure me that my info dumping does not bother them, rather, they love listening to me. It's a warm, fuzzy, and welcoming feeling that every neurodivergent person deserves to feel.

When talking about my special interests with others, I do so because I feel safe in the environment that they have provided for me. I also tend to either infodump or overshare anything to do with my special interest because it excites me so much that I want to share what I know with others in the hopes that they get as excited as I do. It's almost comforting, I suppose, to relish in the things that make me happy. To share it with others is freeing. My tendency to overshare, however, can cause bits of anxiety if I feel that the person I'm infodumping with doesn't show any sort of interest even to listen. That's when I find I crawl back into a shell and keep my interests to myself.

Let me share some of my interests with you. They can be divided into two categories: history and superheroes. I absolutely LOVE history, be it Ancient, South Asian, or Islamic history specifically. I think the reason why I love these strands of history so much is because of the link to my own heritage and faith. It feels liberating to learn more about myself and my people and to increase the love I have for my identity and my faith. Learning, in my eyes, is freedom, and there is nothing I seek more when seeking knowledge. It's also just, straight up interesting. The same applies to Ancient History, which I find incredibly fascinating to dive deep into. Reading about how people before us lived without colonial influence (another interest of mine!) and modern technology is simply just . . . mind-boggling, to be honest, in the best way possible. In relation to this, I love educating myself on social justice issues, which includes studying and understanding colonialism. To me, understanding how my people were treated at the hands of the colonial project is pivotal in shaping my praxis as a teacher, activist, and decent human being.

On the flip side, I adore comics, superheroes and that alike. I enjoy all sorts of media such as books like *The Phoenix King* by Aparna Verma or tv shows like *Moon Knight*; they all entice me with intrigue and the need to know more. It also fuels my imagination and makes me feel refreshed, I've always been like that. Watching an emotional episode of *Demon Slayer*, for example, ignites me with a passion to write something of a similar nature myself to practice my creative writing skills. It's my fuel, my bread and butter. Since I was a kid I always enjoyed relishing in shows like *Power Rangers*, *Winx Club*, and anything similar. I don't exactly know why I loved it so much, I just know that I did. Maybe it was the vibrancy, all of the colours and the cool outfits and costumes and all the fun abilities characters would possess. I just know it filled me with raw joy. Absolute joy, be it childish, but it is pure joy for me. Dopamine. Engaging in a comic, superhero tv show or any sort of fantasy media, be it a book or movie, swallows me in this childish joy that I hold onto so dearly. It's a type of joy that feels like I've just had 5 cups of coffee and I'm going through a caffeine rush. It's bliss and I'll never give it up, not for anybody or anything.

In my experience, I find I become completely unaware of social cues in the 'heat' of the special interest infodump, almost like I become 'lost' in it. This is not necessarily a bad thing, but in rare cases, I might tend to forget to eat, go to the bathroom, or acquire a decent amount of sleep because of my indulgence in my special interest, whether that is me pursuing an activity related to the special interest, talking about the special interest, or being involved in it in some shape or form intensely. It can be unhealthy for me sometimes with the amount I can get lost in the special interest or activity associated with it, but it feels liberating in the moment. It makes me feel like the bits of knowledge I have on abstract concepts that others may not know make me feel like a valuable contributor to growing the understanding of others. Perhaps this is because I am a teacher by profession, but sharing my dedicated interests is a freeing and confidence-boosting experience.

Special schools 🏢

Special schools in the UK cater to students with special educational needs and disabilities (SEND) by offering tailored curricula and resources. However, the term 'special schools' has faced criticism for reinforcing a deficit-based view of neurodivergence, implying separation due to inadequacy. Advocates suggest alternatives like 'inclusive education centres' or 'learning support schools' to emphasise support and adaptability without stigma.

Segregating autistic students in special schools has also been criticised for perpetuating exclusion and ableism, limiting opportunities for inclusion and mutual understanding. This has led to a growing movement towards inclusive education models that integrate neurodivergent students into mainstream settings with appropriate accommodations. Resource-based provision aligns with this approach, offering specialised support within mainstream schools. This approach seeks to balance the benefits of inclusive education – such as social integration and access to a broader curriculum – with targeted support to meet students' needs, reducing the reliance on separate institutions.

Specialist colleges 🏢

These are educational settings in the UK that serve young people aged 16 to 25 with special educational needs and disabilities (SEND) with the aim of bridging educational gaps and boosting employment prospects for young adults. These institutions aim to create an inclusive space by recognising and supporting the varying sensory, communication, and learning styles experienced by neurodivergent students. Their courses often focus on a mix of life skills, vocational training, and academic qualifications. Many specialist colleges will also provide access to speech and language therapy, occupational therapy, counselling, and other targeted support services. This model also often extends to residential options, allowing for a 24-hour learning environment that reinforces personal development, social integration, and skill-building.

Speech and language therapy 🛡

Speech and language therapy is designed to address communication challenges, including those faced by autistic individuals. Traditionally, this therapy has aimed to 'correct' or 'normalise' speech patterns, often through a medical model that pressures neurodivergent people to conform to neurotypical standards. A neurodivergent-affirming approach, however, focuses on empowering authentic self-expression, celebrating and harnessing each person's unique way of communicating. This inclusive approach integrates strategies like augmentative and alternative communication (AAC) and providing adaptations and support for the client's particular learning needs and styles. Such therapies may leverage a person's specific interests to enable the client to unmask, be their authentic self, reduce anxiety, and increase engagement.

Speech dysfluency

Speech dysfluency refers to variations or interruptions in the flow of speaking that differ from neurotypical expectations. The concept recognises that speech is naturally diverse and any interruption – such as stuttering, hesitations, repetitions, or unique rhythms – should be seen as part of the speaker's authentic way of communicating rather than a 'deficit' or something to be 'corrected.' Ultimately, people who experience speech dysfluency require acceptance, respect, and access to spaces that value and support all communication styles. Language should focus on inclusion and genuine listening rather than pressure for 'typical' speech patterns.

Speech-sound difficulties

Speech-sound difficulties refer to challenges in producing specific sounds in typical ways, which can affect the clarity and intelligibility of speech. These issues stem from variations in the coordination of the mouth, tongue, and respiratory muscles and reflect differences in neurological and physical processing. They are unrelated to intellectual ability.

The term 'difficulties' contrasts with the clinical label 'speech-sound disorders,' which frames such differences as deficits requiring treatment. A neurodivergent-affirming perspective values these challenges as natural variations in communication, emphasising support and respect over correction or rejection. Support often includes tailored strategies suited to sensory and learning needs, such as assistive technology, visual aids, or alternative communication methods.

Spoon extending

Spoon extending builds on the spoon theory, which describes the limited daily energy resources – or 'spoons' – available to neurodivergent individuals. While spoon theory emphasises wise allocation of spoons, spoon extending focuses on strategies to replenish or conserve energy. These include rest breaks, sensory regulation techniques, soothing stimming, or pacing systems to prevent burnout.

For example, a person who finds social interactions and crowded spaces particularly draining might use a pacing system by scheduling quieter activities or downtime before and after attending a family gathering. This could include having a sensory-friendly break room available or limiting the duration of social events they commit to. Ultimately, the goal of spoon extending is to create sustainable energy rhythms and prevent prolonged periods of fatigue. By consciously and strategically managing how energy is spent and regained, spoon extending empowers individuals to better navigate daily demands.

Spoon theory

Spoon theory is a metaphor used to illustrate the daily energy limitations often experienced by people with chronic illnesses, disabilities, or neurodivergent identities, including autistic people. It conceptualises energy as a finite resource, represented by spoons. Each task, from getting out of bed to social interactions, 'costs' a certain number of spoons, meaning that a person must carefully manage their spoons to avoid exhaustion or burnout. For neurodivergent individuals, sensory sensitivities, coping with demands, navigating socio-cultural norms and expectations, and dealing with environments designed for neurotypical people can make daily life more 'spoon-depleting.' Unlike many general approaches to fatigue, spoon theory uniquely focuses on self-awareness and self-compassion in managing one's energy levels.

Stimming

'Stimming,' or self-stimulatory behaviour, includes repetitive actions like rocking, fidgeting, flapping, hair twirling, or repeating words. Stimming serves as a crucial tool for self-regulation, helping to manage sensory overload, express emotions, and maintain focus. It should not be viewed as a behaviour needing control or suppression. Autistic people – and anyone else – who can fully embrace their authentic selves will feel free to stim. However, in environments that lack neurodivergent affirmation, masking may occur, leading to significant short- and long-term harm. Some so-called therapies even aim to directly suppress stimming, an approach that is highly damaging.

Educational settings can support autistic individuals by offering quiet zones or sensory-friendly spaces for stimming. These areas provide a safe environment for self-regulation without forcing them to suppress natural coping strategies.

In the workplace, employers can produce an inclusive environment by allowing the use of noise-cancelling headphones, providing access to private spaces for breaks, and training staff to understand and accept neurodivergent behaviours such as stimming. These adjustments help reduce the sensory and social demands placed on autistic employees, enabling them to work more effectively and comfortably.

These approaches empower autistic people by validating their experiences and addressing the real barriers they face rather than enforcing conformity to restrictive norms.

IN MY OWN WORDS: JORIS FOUET

What's the most important thing in your environment right now? Is it your anxiety? Would a slap in the face help?

... It would change the subject for a second.

That's basically what stimming is: a perception that reprioritises your environment.

What's amazing is I can trigger some of those myself!

I have toys, for example. It looks weird: like I'm fidgeting and not paying attention. When, in fact, this is how I engineer hard focus.

It's not that I like it. Rather, it's that in some specific circumstances, it's my only way out. When I get overwhelmed (and neon lights will get me overwhelmed), I feel like I'm spread too thin.

Like everything is tugging at my focus in so many different directions that the only possible outcome is tearing it apart. Unless, obviously, one of them trumps all the others. And when that happens, it grounds me, and from there, I can mount another assault on the rest of it.

The stim can be anything.

Pain works really well. But it is not sustainable.

My best one at the moment is the weirdness of the gyroscopic effect. When I use a heavy fidget spinner, my body can't predict how it behaves. And suddenly, to all the things screaming at me, I can simply say, "hold on a second, you sound important, but this is weirder." And once that pull has been satisfied, I get to decide where I refocus next instead of my environment deciding for me.

The good thing about this one is it has no long-term consequences. I'm just spinning. It just gives me a hit and I can do it again right after.

The tragedy is that I can use drugs for that as well.

And once I get that split second of stimulation, I'm committed to the come down. When all I needed was a distraction.

Strengths-based approach ⚖️ 🛡️

A strengths-based approach focuses on recognising and valuing the unique abilities and potential of each individual, including autistic and other neurodivergent people. It moves away from viewing autism through a lens of deficits or shortcomings, instead highlighting the talents and perspectives neurodivergent individuals bring to their communities.

For example, an educational setting might reframe a student's deep focus on coding, not as a distraction from the curriculum but as an opportunity. Educators could incorporate coding into maths, use it for artistic expression through creative projects, or connect it to historical lessons on technological developments. This approach empowers by embracing diverse ways of thinking, interacting, and processing information.

Adopting the approach has also been shown to boost resilience, social connectedness, self-confidence, and hope. However, it is not always straightforward. Societies that stigmatise or devalue neurodivergence and disability can make its application challenging, and individuals experiencing poor mental health, internalised stigma may find it difficult to embrace their strengths.

Structural stigma 🚫

Structural stigma refers to systemic and institutional discrimination against autistic and other neurodivergent people. It often appears in public policies, organisational practices, and societal norms that disadvantage autistic individuals by embedding biases into systems like healthcare, education, and employment.

The stigma can range from subtle, often unnoticed forms to overt, more easily recognisable discrimination. At its more subtle end, it might involve practices such as educational curricula that fail to represent neurodivergent perspectives or workplace cultures that implicitly favour neurotypical communication styles, thus disadvantaging autistic employees. Or, more overtly, it may involve healthcare systems refusing necessary accommodations, leading to disparities in access and outcomes for autistic patients.

While dismantling structural stigma is challenging, it can be mitigated through autistic-led initiatives and meaningful neurodivergent involvement in shaping policies and practices. Achieving real change requires institutional investment and genuine commitment rather than the tokenistic or tick-box approaches that often undermine efforts towards lasting inclusion and equity.

Stuttering

Stuttering is a speech pattern characterised by disruptions in the flow of speech, such as repetitions, prolonged sounds, or silent blocks where no sound emerges despite an effort to speak. It is a neurological phenomenon rooted in differences in brain function and speech processing, not a psychological issue or defect to be corrected. As such, stuttering should be viewed as a variation in communication and information processing styles.

Around 1% of the global population stutters, with approximately 5% of children experiencing it at some stage, and it is more common in males. Notably, many people who stutter do not experience disruptions while singing. This occurs because singing engages neural pathways for rhythm and melody, which differ from those used in typical speech processing.

Negative social attitudes towards stuttering create barriers, including stigma and misconceptions about intelligence, affecting self-esteem and social participation. Addressing these attitudes is key to creating greater understanding and acceptance of stuttering as a natural variation in communication.

Suicidal ideation

This refers to thoughts or contemplations about ending one's own life. These thoughts can range from fleeting considerations to more detailed planning. Suicidal ideation is not an act itself but a state of mind that can reflect significant distress, despair, or feelings of hopelessness. It is not a sign of weakness but often an indicator that a person feels overwhelmed by their circumstances.

Suicidal ideation is notably higher among autistic people due to the systemic challenges they face, including stigma, isolation, and a lack of understanding from society. The emotional toll of masking and sensory overloads may also contribute.

Support for someone experiencing such thoughts must go beyond offering platitudes. It includes creating an unwaveringly safe, non-judgemental space where they feel heard and validated. Affirming their intrinsic worth and focusing on immediate, practical adjustments to reduce stressors – whether by addressing sensory environments or removing pressures to mask – can be transformative. Professional mental health support rooted in neurodiversity-affirming practices can also be crucial.

Access to peer support, where one can connect with others who understand their experiences, can offer a vital lifeline. For those encountering such thoughts, recognising that no situation is permanent and seeking trusted allies to share the burden can be an important first step. Every life holds inherent value, and a culture of acceptance and connection can help mitigate the despair often hidden behind these thoughts.

IN MY OWN WORDS: WILLIAM VANDERPUYE

From a personal experience, suicidal ideation is a secondary instinct that is triggered by adversity, however small or meaningless. A nasty phone call, an embarrassing memory, a parking fine, a failed exam, financial problems. These are instances that have triggered thoughts that I would be better off dead.

That does not mean that I want to die. It does not necessarily mean that I will act on it. On the other hand, it does not necessarily mean that I will not act on it. Most people who have suicidal ideation do not want to die.

I do not see it as a sign of weakness but as a sign that I have been strong for too long, that I have pretended to be fine for too long, prioritising other people's feelings at the expense of my own until I cannot take it anymore.

Prior to embarking on my social work degree, I had to undergo fitness to practice screenings. I was put through particularly high levels of scrutiny because of my neurodivergence. I was given a lengthy questionnaire by my university and a form to be given to my GP to fill. The process was so stressful that I felt it was the end of the road for me, that they would come back to me saying I would not be allowed to pursue the programme. In desperation, my brain began to look for an escape. An escape from this cruel world with cruel and oppressive rules that work for some and does not work for others. Many a times, I have felt like these 'others,' and this would continue to torture me until I die naturally within the next 40 to 50 years … or I could put myself out of my misery by …

Often, I catch myself subconsciously or instinctively making plans and thinking about suicide when things do not go to plan and life hurts. I then make a conscious effort to stop myself, think positive thoughts, exercise, listen to music, distract myself, read a comic book, do something that does not entail boredom or tedium, take a break from working hard and allow myself to heal. Because suicidal ideation bruises me. It is like self-harming to my soul.

There is something that draws me to it to help me deal with the pain of life. That is why I practice self-care; I avoid the company of critics and places where I am tolerated in favour of places where I feel celebrated.

I have been prescribed talking therapy and medication, all of which have played a part in the regulation of my emotions. For a long time, I have not had the urge to give up on life, and I have responded positively to treatment. If a loved one experiences suicidal ideation, take it seriously. They need love and understanding, room to express themselves and a listening ear. They do not need to hear how privileged they are or how selfish they are to consider suicide. They do not need to be taken on a guilt trip because of how their children and partner would feel. These will only worsen the situation. They need a listening ear. They would probably come up with the appropriate solution given the right conditions: a supportive environment and an active non-judgemental and empathetic listener.

Sunflower lanyard ⚖️ 🛡️

The sunflower lanyard is a green lanyard with a bright yellow sunflower pattern. It signals that the wearer has a hidden disability and may need extra assistance, patience, or understanding. Gatwick Airport in the UK first introduced the scheme in 2016 to improve accessibility and create more inclusive environments for individuals with non-visible disabilities.

The initiative has expanded internationally to airports, public venues, and organisations in countries including the USA, Australia, Canada, and India. In 2023, the world's longest lanyard, representing 867 hidden disabilities, was displayed at Liverpool Football Club's Anfield stadium to symbolise the scheme's global impact. That same year, Brazil adopted the sunflower symbol as its national emblem for hidden disabilities, marking the occasion by projecting the sunflower onto the Christ the Redeemer statue.

IN MY OWN WORDS: WILLIAM VANDERPUYE

I had just opened my front door and taken a few maiden steps into my street, which was quieter than usual. I am not a very outgoing person, so being confined to the comfort of my home for any considerable amount of time was a godsend – as long as my family had everything they needed. In this instance, however, we needed food. This was the first lockdown of the COVID-19 pandemic, which bore the bittersweet resemblance to an Orwellian era where everyone's movement was tracked and venturing outdoors was only permitted if it was absolutely necessary. The queue outside my local supermarket was reminiscent of the communist period in a movie I once watched, where citizens had to queue for their daily rations. Social distancing made the queue even longer. Then something caught my eye: a green lanyard with sunflowers worn by a lady in front of me. I had seen a similar lanyard a few weeks earlier, but I thought nothing of it. This time, curiosity got the best of me, and I researched it on my phone. It turned out to be an indicator of a hidden disability, which would prompt staff to enquire whether the wearer needed assistance.

I grew up in Accra, Ghana, during the 1980s and 1990s, a time and place where one's disability was concealed due to stigma. In my community, disability was seen as a curse from God, a punishment for sin, or even something evil brought by the devil. Families avoided any association with disability because it was believed to tarnish their reputation. Autism and neurodivergence were not understood, and individuals who presented differently from the norm were ridiculed and ostracised. Terms like 'abodamfo' (mad people) were thrown around, and children mocked those who struggled. I often saw people with severe mental illnesses roaming the streets of Accra, naked or in dirt-covered rags, eating from bins, their hair matted. No one asked how they ended up like this or whether they needed help; instead, they were seen as objects of derision. This shaped my childhood understanding of mental illness and disability – not as something to support but as something to fear or reject.

When I returned to Ghana as a teenager after spending part of my childhood in France, where I had learned to mask my differences, I still couldn't escape ridicule. People could see through my masking. My fixation on rocks and stones, my struggles with social interaction – these differences were not tolerated. I was given derogatory names, and even as an adult, I've seen how these attitudes persist. For many, the focus remains on how to 'fix' or 'pray away' disability rather than embrace acceptance.

When I was formally diagnosed as autistic in the UK, some friends and family welcomed it, saying, "You've always been you, nothing has changed." But for others, it was a struggle. They rejected the diagnosis outright, claiming autism didn't exist in Africans. Some were embarrassed by my openness about being autistic, urging me to keep silent for the sake of the family's reputation. But I refused to stay quiet. Advocacy became my way of challenging the stigma I grew up with and helping others understand that neurodivergence isn't something to hide.

The sunflower lanyard felt like a game changer. With it, I could make a statement without saying a word. It became a silent campaign for acceptance, even on days when I had no energy to explain myself. I eventually received my first lanyard from the CEO of Autistic Inclusive Meets, which I wore with pride. It highlighted both my strengths and my vulnerabilities, helping people understand when I was distressed or triggered, encouraging them to be more patient and compassionate.

While the sunflower lanyard is widely recognised in the UK, its visibility abroad is limited. On a trip to Ghana for six weeks, I realised that mine was the only sunflower lanyard I saw. No one asked about it, and its purpose was completely unrecognised. This experience reminded me of the long road ahead in challenging stigma in my community, where attitudes towards disability are still deeply rooted in the religious and medical models.

Despite this, I remain hopeful. I've shared my experiences with the lanyard in my workplace's Hidden Disabilities campaign, on podcasts, and on social media. For me, it is more than a practical tool – it's a symbol of visibility and acceptance, a small but powerful step towards a world that understands and embraces hidden disabilities.

Synaesthesia

Synaesthesia is a neurological phenomenon affecting 1–4% of people, where stimulation of one sensory pathway triggers automatic, involuntary experiences in another. It might involve seeing colours when hearing music, associating words with tastes, or sensing textures with sounds. For example, someone who experiences chromesthesia – a type of synaesthesia – might consistently see vibrant bursts of colour whenever they hear specific musical notes; imagine hearing a violin's high note and visualising a vivid flash of blue. Grapheme-colour synaesthesia, one of the most common forms, links specific colours to letters or numbers, such as the letter 'A' always appearing red or the number '5' green. Synaesthetic perceptions can also be highly consistent over time; if a sound evokes a specific colour, it will reliably do so in every instance. This consistency can enhance memory and creativity, often helping synaesthetes excel in artistic or creative pursuits.

Tactile sense

The tactile sense refers to how individuals perceive physical contact with their environment. For autistic people, neurological differences can intensify or dull these sensory experiences. Heightened sensitivity may lead to discomfort from light touches, clothing tags, or certain textures, often causing distress or an urgent need to avoid the stimuli. Removing tags, using seamless clothing, or choosing soft, non-abrasive fabrics can help. Conversely, some autistic individuals seek tactile input, finding regulation through deep pressure or specific types of touch. Weighted blankets, deep-pressure massage, or compression garments can provide relief and reduce anxiety or sensory overload. Tactile processing shapes how neurodivergent individuals engage with the physical world, underscoring the need for personalised sensory support.

Theory of mind

The term 'theory of mind' refers to the capacity to understand that others have their own thoughts, feelings, and perspectives, which may differ from one's own. This is often incorrectly framed as a perceived deficit among autistic people, with the view they are unable to recognise and predict other peoples' mental states, leading to challenges in social interactions. This notion, however, is both reductionist and outdated, and it fails to appreciate the diversity of autistic cognitive styles and the unique ways they engage in social reciprocity.

For example, autistic people may communicate in direct ways, valuing honesty and detail, which some non-autistic people misinterpret as a lack of empathy or social awareness. However, this is simply a different way of connecting and communicating. Some autistic people may also develop deep bonds through shared interests or routines, demonstrating their unique approach to reciprocity and connection. Rather than a deficit, this highlights how autistic cognitive styles promote social engagement on their own terms, showing that many autistic people can and do develop effective ways of understanding others, even if these differ from non-autistic norms.

Thermoceptive sense 💬

The thermoceptive sense refers to the body's ability to detect and process temperature variations, playing a key role in maintaining core body temperature and ensuring physical comfort. This sense operates by perceiving warmth, cold, and shifts in ambient temperature, prompting responses like seeking warmth when cold or sweating when hot. Sensory receptors in the skin and the brain's interpretation of these signals regulate this process.

For some neurodivergent people, thermoception may differ, leading to heightened or reduced responses to temperature changes. This is referred to as thermosensitivity. This can result in behaviours like seeking specific environments for sensory comfort or avoiding certain temperatures.

Tickertape synaesthesia 💬

Tickertape synaesthesia is a cognitive phenomenon often reported by autistic people, in which their thoughts and perceptions feel as though they are constantly flowing, like a mental stream of words or images scrolling across a screen. This involuntary phenomenon may involve verbal or visual information and can feel overwhelming in its detail or speed. For instance, an autistic person might listen to a conversation while simultaneously 'seeing' the spoken words spelled out in their mind, as though they were subtitles. This can create intense focus but may also make it challenging to keep up with the pace of the discussion. This mental tickertape can also extend to environments with overlapping conversations, where a stream of visualised words from different speakers appear in one's mind, making it difficult and exhausting to focus, particularly in crowded or noisy settings. Many autistic individuals describe it as 'living with subtitles.'

While many neurotypical individuals might also have an internal monologue or visual thinking, the experience of tickertape synaesthesia is often more vivid, persistent, and consuming for autistic individuals. It can be a source of creativity and insight and aid with spelling and language acquisition, but it can also a challenge, particularly in situations that demand immediate responses or multitasking.

Tourette's 💬

Tourette's is a neurological identity primarily characterised by involuntary motor and vocal tics – sudden movements or sounds made repeatedly and often without warning. Tics vary in complexity, from blinking or throat clearing to more intricate movements or phrases. While often stereotyped by coprolalia (involuntary swearing or taboo speech), this type of tic is rare and not representative of most cases. Tourette's typically emerges in childhood and frequently co-occurs with other neurodivergent identities.

Tic severity and type often fluctuate over time, influenced by factors such as stress, fatigue, or joy, with safe, neurodivergent-affirming social support and spaces particularly effective in reducing tic frequency.

It is vital to approach Tourette's without stigma, focusing instead on acceptance and understanding rather than suppression or 'normalisation' of tics. Creating inclusive environments tailored to individuals' needs ensures that tics are recognised as part of the person's authentic self and do not diminish their worth.

Transitions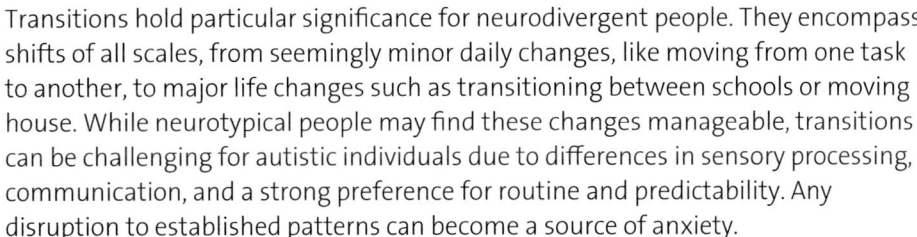

Transitions hold particular significance for neurodivergent people. They encompass shifts of all scales, from seemingly minor daily changes, like moving from one task to another, to major life changes such as transitioning between schools or moving house. While neurotypical people may find these changes manageable, transitions can be challenging for autistic individuals due to differences in sensory processing, communication, and a strong preference for routine and predictability. Any disruption to established patterns can become a source of anxiety.

Successfully navigating transitions involves thoughtful planning, clear communication, and the use of supportive strategies like visual schedules or sensory-friendly environments. Involvement in planning can help reduce stress by enabling the individual through autonomy, control, and respect. Moreover, strategies tailored to individual sensory needs and executive functioning challenges are essential for minimising the overwhelm that transitions can provoke. Proper support ensures these changes are gradual and manageable, enabling a sense of safety during periods of uncertainty.

Trauma

Trauma is a deeply distressing experience that disrupts an individual's sense of safety, trust, and identity. For neurodivergent individuals, trauma often carries heightened impacts due to several overlapping factors. These include higher rates of adverse experiences like abuse, discrimination, and exclusion; chronic stress from navigating neurotypical expectations; sensory sensitivities that amplify traumatic experiences; and the cumulative effects of societal ableism and stigma. Communication differences can make it harder to express distress or seek help, creating cycles of overwhelm and isolation. The pathologising lens of the medical model often adds to this harm by framing neurodivergent traits as inherently problematic.

Healing requires neurodivergent-affirming approaches that validate individual experiences. Autistic-led, trauma-informed care is essential, recognising both the challenges and strengths of neurodivergent individuals. Prioritising safe environments, honouring sensory needs, and building resilience through acceptance rather than conformity are key to recovery.

Tribunals ⚖️

Tribunals are formal bodies designed to resolve disputes outside traditional court systems. For autistic and other neurodivergent individuals, they can play for a vital role in addressing issues such as discrimination, education needs, and social care provision. These forums are meant to offer accessible, specialised adjudication by panels with expertise in the relevant field.

The UK's Special Educational Needs and Disability (SEND) Tribunal is a key example, particularly in education. In the 2021/2022 academic year, 7,200 appeals were registered – a 29% increase from the previous year. Many of these cases involved autism-specific disputes, reflecting the persistent challenges families face in securing appropriate educational support for their autistic children.

Despite being designed for accessibility, tribunals often pose challenges for autistic individuals and their families. Procedural complexity, unfamiliar settings, and the adversarial nature of proving entitlement to services can be overwhelming and retraumatising. While tribunals are intended to be less intimidating than traditional courts, robust advocacy and legal support are often necessary to help autistic individuals navigate these systems and ensure their needs are fully understood and addressed.

Trichotillomania

Trichotillomania refers to the compulsive self-regulatory urge to pull out one's hair. The repetitive, highly tactile nature of hair-pulling may offer a form of sensory anchoring – a way to ground oneself when other sensory and emotional regulatory systems are overwhelmed.

Rather than focusing on behaviour suppression, support should focus primarily on identifying the underlying sensory needs and environmental triggers that are overwhelming the individual. Developing alternative, safer regulation strategies that honour the individual's neurological makeup are also encouraged. A compassionate, neurodivergent-affirming approach that works with, rather than against, the individual's need to pull hair during overwhelm is vital.

Triggers 🌿

Triggers are stimuli, either external or internal, that can precipitate intense physiological, emotional, or behavioural responses in neurodivergent individuals.

For autistic people and others, triggers often stem from sensory inputs that overwhelm neural systems, disruptions to routines, or social dynamics that impose heavy cognitive demands.

The manifestation of triggers varies significantly across individuals and contexts. While one person might experience acute distress from fluorescent lighting or unexpected touch, another might find certain social expectations or transitions particularly challenging. These responses are not merely preferences or inconveniences – they represent genuine neurological reactions that can lead to overwhelming anxiety, sensory overload, or complete shutdown. Recognising the neurological basis of triggers reframes them as valid responses, not oversensitivities, and highlights the diverse ways neurodivergent individuals process and experience the world.

Triple empathy

The triple empathy concept extends the idea of the double empathy problem, which recognises that communication challenges between autistic and non-autistic individuals stem from differences in perspectives and cultural understandings rather than social deficits. 'Triple empathy' builds on this by highlighting how unique professional cultures, particularly within healthcare and other institutional settings, add a third dimension to these communication gaps. This can lead to additional misunderstandings when autistic people interact with healthcare professionals due to differing cultural norms, jargon, and practices. This subsequently further increases the risk of anxiety and sensory overload and can lead to feelings of helplessness, loss of autonomy, and withdrawal. Addressing these issues requires healthcare institutions to train staff in neurodivergent communication styles, simplify jargon, and ensure sensory-friendly environments. Collaborative, patient-centred care, clear and flexible communication strategies, and involving autistic individuals in service design can further bridge these divides and enable more inclusive, effective care.

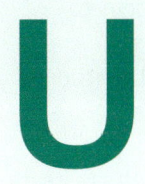

Unintentional stigma

The term 'unintentional stigma' describes biases, stereotypes, and behaviours that harm neurodivergent individuals, often without the person enacting them realising the impact. It stems from deeply ingrained societal norms and assumptions that frame autism through a medical lens, as something to 'fix' or as inherently 'deficient.' It is reflected in seemingly minor acts, like a teacher praising a child for 'not acting autistic today,' or a healthcare professional assuming an autistic adult is incapable of understanding their own needs. Language plays a role too – assumptions about a lack of empathy or social skills strip autistic people of their humanity and individuality. Social behaviours grounded in ignorance, like excluding someone from a conversation because their communication style is different, may not be malicious but still leave lasting scars.

Unintentional stigma fuels misconceptions, reinforcing a world that sees autistic individuals as 'other' and creating barriers to belonging. These moments, small as they seem, can accumulate into a profound sense of alienation. Imagine an autistic adult who is endlessly commended for masking their traits but never for their authentic self. Consider a parent whose well-meaning friends suggest 'cures' for their autistic child, unknowingly invalidating their child's identity. Such examples illustrate how unintentional stigma perpetuates marginalisation, even when borne from care or goodwill.

United Nations Convention on the Rights of Persons With Disabilities (CRPD)

The UN Convention on the Rights of Persons with Disabilities, created in 2006, is a landmark treaty ensuring equal rights and dignity for disabled people. It stresses social inclusion, accessibility, and full participation in all aspects of life, guided by principles of respect for dignity, non-discrimination, inclusion, and equal opportunity.

The CRPD urges governments to pass laws banning discrimination against disabled individuals, including autistic people, in employment, healthcare, education,

DOI: 10.4324/9781003477297-18

and public access. It redefines disability using a social model, shifting focus to societal barriers rather than individual limitations. This shift champions empowerment and self-determination while addressing structural and attitudinal challenges faced by disabled communities.

As the first human rights treaty of the 21st century, the CRPD was also the fastest negotiated, concluding in just four years. In 2007, 82 countries signed on the first day, a record for any UN Convention. This overwhelming support reflects a global commitment to inclusion and dignity for disabled people.

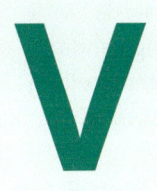

Vestibular sense

The vestibular sense plays a key role in enabling balance, movement coordination, and spatial orientation. This system works alongside proprioception – the sense of body position and movement – to help maintain physical control and awareness. Together, they enable smooth and regulated actions like standing, walking, and everyday movements. Many autistic and neurodivergent individuals experience differences in their vestibular and proprioceptive senses, affecting balance, gait, or physical activities. Consider an individual whose vestibular system interprets swings as exhilarating one day and terrifying the next or someone who navigates crowded spaces with the constant sensation of being on a shifting boat.

These variations often intersect with dyspraxia, a motor coordination difference that can make planning and executing movements more challenging. Supportive environments with sensory-friendly resources – such as balance boards, swings, weighted blankets, or textured paths – can help neurodivergent individuals regulate their sensory input and movement in ways that feel safe and empowering.

Victimisation

Victimisation involves targeting individuals for mistreatment, often based on their identity or characteristics, causing harm or disadvantage. This issue profoundly affects neurodivergent communities, where autistic people are especially vulnerable, experiencing bullying and discrimination at significantly higher rates than their neurotypical peers.

It can take many forms, including exclusion, social ostracism, workplace inequities, and systemic discrimination. Intersectional identities further intensify the risk, layering multiple forms of stigma. Institutional structures can also exacerbate victimisation, embedding ableist assumptions and policies that undervalue neurodivergent needs and enforce conformity to neurotypical norms at great personal cost.

Consider this example: an autistic employee in a high-pressure workplace is repeatedly reprimanded for not maintaining eye contact during meetings and for avoiding unstructured social interactions, such as team lunches. Despite excelling in their role and delivering results beyond expectations, they are perceived as disengaged, unfriendly, or even uncooperative because of these neurodivergent traits. Efforts to explain their needs are dismissed as excuses, and their manager questions their 'cultural fit.' Over time, they are passed over for promotions, excluded from key projects, and subjected to gossip about their 'difficult' personality. Ultimately, the stress becomes unbearable, and they resign – not because of incompetence but because the environment systematically denies their right to exist authentically.

Virtual reality

Virtual reality (VR) immerses users in digitally simulated environments through interactive sensory experiences. Unlike passive media, VR encourages active engagement via devices like headsets, gloves, or controllers. Its uses extend beyond entertainment to education, therapy, and accessibility tools for neurodivergent individuals.

For example, VR is increasingly being used to support mental health, offering unique therapeutic opportunities for those facing challenges such as anxiety, depression, and PTSD. Immersive experiences can transport users to calming environments, teach coping mechanisms, and provide tailored sensory experiences that reduce anxiety. It may also help with social rehearsal, unmasking, connection-building, mindfulness, and sensory exploration.

However, VR must be designed with care to avoid overstimulation, particularly for autistic users, and to manage the risk of encountering unfriendly and stigmatising interactions online. Safe online spaces are essential, with strong moderation and community guidelines that create respectful and supportive environments, so neurodivergent individuals can explore and connect without fear of negative experiences.

Visual processing disorder

The term 'visual processing disorder' refers to neurological differences affecting how the brain interprets visual information rather than issues with vision itself. This can manifest as difficulty distinguishing shapes, such as struggling to tell the difference between a circle and an oval, and recognising familiar objects, such as finding it hard to identify a friend in a crowd due to an overload of visual information or challenges in processing facial features in complex environments. It can also impact spatial awareness, such as judging distances, which might make tasks like climbing stairs or playing sports challenging, as well as interpreting visual sequences, such as reading. It is worth noting that these differences are not indicative of intelligence or overall cognitive ability but rather reflect a unique way of processing and interacting with visual stimuli. With appropriate understanding and support, individuals with these differences can navigate their environments and tasks effectively.

Visual sense

The visual sense pertains to the ability to process and interpret visual stimuli from the environment through sight, a key sensory system. For neurodivergent people, there may be visual processing that result in a non-typical experience of vision. For example, heightened visual processing may lead to exceptional attention to detail, pattern recognition, or visual memory, offering strengths in fields like art or engineering. However, these differences can also contribute to sensory sensitivities or visual overwhelm, particularly in environments with high visual clutter or rapid changes. This variability underscores the importance of tailoring environments to individual visual processing needs, such as minimising sensory overload or creating visually structured settings.

Voiced empathy

This refers to the process of actively communicating genuine understanding and care in a way that deeply resonates with the other person. Unlike traditional assumptions that define empathy as merely feeling or mirroring another's emotional state, voiced empathy centres on intentional, clear, and direct expression of support, often shaped by the unique communication needs and preferences of neurodivergent individuals.

For example, an autistic person may express their empathy by offering detailed advice or a practical solution rather than a typical reassuring phrase. They might also demonstrate voiced empathy by explicitly acknowledging the other person's feelings, such as saying, "I've been reading about what you're going through, and I'm here if you'd like to share more or need any support." This direct expression conveys genuine care and validates the other person's experience through clear and intentional communication. Conversely, they may also communicate empathy through focused listening, which can be profound yet different from expected non-speaking cues like facial expressions or touch.

This further highlights that many autistic people possess profound empathy but may express it differently, requiring non-autistic people to adapt and learn to receive and convey empathy across neurotypes.

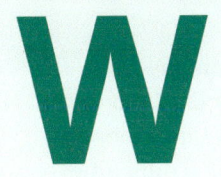

Wearables

Wearables are devices and technologies designed to support sensory, communication, well-being, and daily living needs for autistic and neurodivergent individuals. These can include sensory aids like noise-cancelling headphones to reduce sensory overload and assistive tools such as smartwatches. Augmented reality glasses, resembling regular eyewear or contact lenses, are likely to become more common and can assist with recognising faces (useful for prosopagnosia), remembering names (useful for anomic aphasia), and enhancing social communication.

Smart clothing, such as adjustable compression vests, provides sensory regulation and comfort, while haptic wristbands and emotion-sensing wearables help detect stress or anxiety, benefiting those with interoception differences. Jewellery, glasses, gloves, and other wearable technologies support sensory and communication needs while respecting individuality. It is also important that ethical development in the wearables field prioritises user-led design that celebrates and supports neurodivergent identity rather than trying to change it.

Wider autism community

The wider autism community includes everyone who supports or engages with autistic people, such as family, friends, educators, healthcare professionals, allies, and advocates, whether autistic or not. At its best, this community creates a network of support, understanding, and mutual respect. While the diversity within this broad group can lead to different, and sometimes problematic, perspectives on autism, the shared aim should be to centre the voices and needs of autistic people themselves, creating a society rooted in acceptance and belonging.

It is vital to recognise that autistic parents, siblings, and friends also have unique lived experiences that enrich this collective. Though challenges, such as stigma, may exist within some segments, there remains an overarching potential for the wider autism community to build bridges of empathy, learning, and collaboration, reinforcing the message that everyone's contributions can lead to a more inclusive and respectful society for autistic people.

Williams syndrome

Williams syndrome is a rare genetic condition caused by a deletion on chromosome 7, giving rise to distinct neurological and physical traits. Individuals with this condition often have unique facial features, cardiovascular challenges such as supravalvular aortic stenosis (a narrowing of the aorta), and difficulties with spatial reasoning. At the same time, they frequently possess exceptional verbal abilities, musical talent, social engagement, and empathy, paired with a strong desire to form connections with others. Their musical aptitude is often associated with hyperacusis, a heightened sensitivity to specific frequencies of sound.

Societal norms, which often prioritise conformity and rigid expectations, can fail to recognise the unique ways individuals with Williams syndrome interact, express themselves, or approach education and work. For example, their openness and eagerness to engage socially might be misunderstood as overly familiar or inappropriate in certain settings. Similarly, traditional education systems, which often focus on standardised approaches, may struggle to adapt to their distinct learning styles. By creating inclusive spaces that celebrate their strengths and embrace their individuality, society can offer them the opportunity to thrive as their authentic selves.